HEALTHY CHILDREN

A Guide for Child Care

Coralie Mathews

MACLENNAN+PETTY
SYDNEY • PHILADELPHIA • LONDON

First published 2001

MacLennan & Petty Pty Limited
Suite 405, 152 Bunnerong Road, Eastgardens, NSW 2036 Australia

National Library of Australia
Cataloguing-in-Publication data:

Mathews, Coralie
Healthy children: a guide for child care
Bibliography
Includes index

ISBN 0 86433 159 2

1. Children – Health and hygiene. 2. Child care – Health aspects.
3. Children – Nutrition. I. Title.
613.0432
Illustrations by Carolyn Brooks
Cover photographs by Theona Poteris, Kandid Kids Photography
Cover design by Pamela Horsnell, Juno Creative Services
Printed and bound in Australia

CONTENTS

FOREWORD

A HUNDRED YEARS ago, around the time of Federation in Australia, the health status of young children was of enormous concern. Infant mortality rates were over 100 per thousand infants born, ie more than one in ten babies would die before their first birthday, mainly from gastroenteritis and other infections.

The conditions in which families lived in all States of Australia, particularly in the main cities, were overcrowded and unhygienic. Fresh water was often contaminated and food rarely nourishing. Fewer than 60% of mothers breastfed their babies. Those that did had ten to twenty times lower rates of death in their infants! The public health leaders of the day, influenced by measures in the United Kingdom and France but without specific knowledge about the organisms causing gastroenteritis, started to implement change.

Over the next 20 to 30 years they must have been immensely satisfied to observe the dramatic falls in infant and child deaths as a result of their policies. These *community* interventions were improved living conditions, alleviation of poverty, education of girls (future mothers), better nutrition (particularly encouraging breastfeeding) and home visiting programs for all new mothers.

It was only later that antibiotics and vaccination kicked in as major preventive strategies.

At the beginning of the 21st century in spite of our wealth and knowledge we are faced with epidemics of complex diseases and psychosocial health problems in our families, children and teenagers. Adverse social and environmental factors are stronger than the drugs and interventions that we have at our disposal to treat these problems. With incomplete knowledge of the specific causal pathways, public health leaders also need to respond to ensure future healthy children.

Providing enriched and healthy early environments for our children may well be the most powerful tool we have.

This book, *Healthy Children: A Guide for Child Care* by Coralie Mathews, has the potential to make a significant contribution to this response. By addressing the social, emotional, physical and preventive health needs of children in childcare it provides information and strategies for childcare workers and parents. Those who read it will be better equipped to lead the charge to improve the environments to grow healthy children.

I am impressed with the breadth and depth of this book. Nothing has been left out. It is an extremely thorough exposition of all of the aspects of physical and social development of children and their needs from the antenatal period through to adolescence. As well, it summarises the broad range of modern diseases, conditions and problems that children experience, and outlines known risk factors and possible preventive strategies to enable appropriate interventions.

Embedded throughout the knowledgeable pages and chapters of this book are excellent little vignettes and case studies, which really bring home the issues that are being addressed in the more academic text around them. They have been used extremely well to illustrate the problems that face many families who are contemplating childcare, or who have children with special needs or who are just trying to bring up children in today's tough world. It seems to me that it has the right mix of both scholarship and pragmatism, with an excellent bibliography at the end of each section for those students who wish to pursue subjects in greater depth. Being a student text it also guides students at the end of each chapter to do some further study or investigation of their own to increase the usefulness of the book.

I was extremely pleased to be asked to write the foreword of this important book but until I had read it I wasn't aware of how powerful an effect I believe it will have. I look forward to observing its success.

Fiona Stanley
AC MBBS MSc MD FFPHM FAFPHM FRACP FRACOG FASSA HonDSc
Director, TVW Telethon Institute for Child Health Research, Perth
The Variety Club Professor of Paediatrics, The University of Western Australia

ACKNOWLEDGMENTS

THIS BOOK OWES much to many people. It is dedicated to the Child Care/Early Childhood Education students of the Northern Territory University and it is this group that I first thank. I thank them for their frank friendliness, their liveliness, their interest, for their humour in late evening classes when we had all worked a long hot day. Most of all I thank them for what they taught me. One of the real joys of teaching is that you learn so much and my teachers were wise in so many ways and generous in sharing that wisdom. I especially thank the Indigenous students for their patient teaching and their willingness to share their experiences, their families and their culture.

I thank the Northern Territory University for allowing me professional development leave to kick-start the writing and Dr Brian Devlin (then Dean of Education) for his support. I am forever grateful to my colleagues in the Faculty of Education at NT University for the right degree of cynicism and hope at appropriate times. My Early Childhood colleagues lived through various stages of the manuscript together with changing curricula, major university structural changes and their own post-graduate studies. Through all this their support was unstinting.

The child care staff of Darwin, Palmerston and the surrounding areas were always welcoming and shared with me both joys and woes. And the childen . . . how can I thank the children who questioned and chatted and told me everybody's names . . . ?

The staff of Menzies School of Health Research were also very helpful and gave much encouragement.

The staff, families and children at Bruce Ridge Early Childhood Centre were so welcoming when I arrived in Canberra. I am grateful for them allowing me to share the children's activities and to photograph the children at play.

I must also thank the Academic Unit of General Practice and Community Care at the Canberra Clinical School for making a major job change such a pleasant experience. Their interest in my writing was much appreciated.

Many people gave time to reviewing the manuscript and made thoughtful and constructive comments which were much valued and appreciated.

And to John, wise in different ways to the students, who stayed supportive and clear-sighted through it all, thank you.

Coralie Mathews
Canberra

Some parts of Chapters 8 and 9 are adapted from training materials copyright to the Australian National Training Authority and used here with their permission.

PREFACE

THIS TEXT IS primarily for trainees, Certificate and Diploma in Children's Services students, and for staff already employed in child-care settings. It has been written for students in the Vocational Education and Training sector, although Higher Education early childhood education students might find some sections useful.

The wide range of topics covered will give students a broad understanding of each subject. Those wishing to extend their knowledge about a particular topic would need to explore a specialist text on that subject.

The aim of the text is to serve as an adjunct to the National Child Care Competencies. It does not set out to be a learning package but rather to provide the underpinning knowledge needed to achieve the Competencies. Links from each chapter to the Competencies are listed in the Appendix.

The text is also intended to extend the learner's own general knowledge of health matters. Child-care professionals are advocates for children's rights, and good health is one of the basic rights of any child. Knowledge of health and related issues allows the child-care professional to have a more comprehensive understanding of how good health can be achieved for themselves, for the children in their care, and for the families of those children. It is hoped that this text will assist students to gain this knowledge by providing accurate information and by using case studies to translate this information into practice in a child-care setting.

Children come to child care as part of a family, from different cultures and with different values, histories and experiences. The diversity of family life is exciting and a cause for celebration, yet we should not forget that there are human needs for physical, social and emotional health that are common to all.

Section 1

The first section of the text looks at child health and the community. Contraception is included, as planning children is a major factor in good health both in Australia and in developing countries. Women and their partners have a right to have accurate information about contraception. A children's service is a community resource that will provide advice (for both parents and staff) about where health services (including family planning) can be obtained. Student health is considered and information about the prevention of STDs is included.

A knowledge of fetal development and the importance of ante-natal care is a prerequisite to a real understanding of the neonate and infant and his/her needs. Similarly an knowledge of the birth process gives an understanding of the family and the young baby.

Caring for children and understanding their physical and other needs is enhanced if the caregiver is familiar with the structure and function of the body. An appreciation of normal growth patterns and the importance of monitoring growth and development is an essential aspect of maintaining health and preventing disease in children.

Section 2

This section examines the health needs of a child within a child-care setting. It includes the hazards to health of infection, poor nutrition, accidents, illness and child abuse.

There is a real risk of increased infections in long-day care, especially among the under-2-year-olds. A basic knowledge of microbiology helps the student understand the reasons why these infections occur. This understanding makes it easier for the caregiver to prevent (or at least to minimise) the spread of infection in a child-care setting.

Health and hygiene education starts when children are young. This can happen through the planning of developmentally appropriate activities so that care routines are extended to be valuable learning experiences for the infant and child.

The integration of health routines into the wider program of activities provided by the child-care setting is important. Health routines have often, in the past, been seen as things that have to be done but which take a child away from play and the important business of their learning. Sensitively done, health routines can be part of play and enhance rather than detract from learning.

Coralie Mathews
May 2000

SECTION 1

Child Health and the Community

CHAPTER 1

Introduction to health

IT COULD BE asked why, in a country such as Australia, are health concerns an issue? Why do students in child-care and early-childhood education courses need to complete modules in health studies? Why are the causes of poor health sometimes misunderstood and the very concept of health itself often debated?

What is health?

Many people think that health is being free of physical illness. However this is only one of the many aspects that makes up a healthy person. Health includes the physical, mental, spiritual and social wellbeing of children, their families and the whole community.

The World Health Organization (WHO) describes health as:

> A state of complete physical, mental and social well-being, and not merely the absence of disease or infirmity. The extension to all peoples of the benefits of medical, physiological and related knowledge is essential to the fullest attainment of health. Informed opinion and active co-operation on the part of the public are of the utmost importance in the improvement of the health of the people.
>
> (WHO, Alma Ata 1978)

This definition emphasises the positive aspects that make up health. The absence of disease is important, but alone it is not enough. A child may be physically healthy with no apparent disease, but be withdrawn and not join in the activities in the child-care setting. It could be that there is some disruption to the family. A well-loved grandparent may have died, a parent may have lost a job, the family may have moved, or a parent may be in hospital. Any disruption to the family is likely to affect the health and wellbeing of the child.

The WHO definition of health also states that knowledge of medical, physiological and related topics is important for improving health. People should be well informed in matters relating to health issues in order to be able to make decisions about their own health and the health of the community. In the past, one of the criticisms of health professionals (often directed at doctors) was that health information was held by the doctors and not given to the community. Fortunately, this situation is changing and more people are gaining an understanding of both personal and community health issues.

Early childhood caregivers and educators work closely with both children and their families. They are in a position to assist with giving 'related knowledge' and extending 'informed opinion' which will benefit not only the health of the children but also the community as a whole. To do this child-care professionals need a broad understanding of child and family health.

The Australian Health Ministers' Advisory Council (AHMAC) policy paper on *The Health of Young Australians* (1995) recognises the importance of this wider definition of health and states that:

> The health of children and young people is influenced by a broad range of family, social, educational, environmental, economic and biological factors; . . .

and

> Health and well-being, as distinct from the narrower concept of absence of illness, is best achieved by attention to a number of stages and levels of care which focus on improved health outcomes. These include health promotion; prevention; early intervention; access to appropriate and affordable services through the strengthening of primary health care; and the maintenance of high quality treatment services for injury, illness and disabilities . . .

and

> Consumer participation in decision making and co-operation between relevant agencies of government, health professionals, non-government organisations and the community are essential to this approach.
>
> (AHMAC 1995)

Stages and levels of care

Primary health care

Primary health care is the health service that people first attend when seeking attention for health concerns. Most primary health care services are available in the community and provide a broad-based range of services. Health promotion and education, together with preventive services, are found at this level. Community health centres, which monitor the health of babies, children and their families, are an essential primary health care preventive service. A community health service or a family doctor also provide primary health care.

Much emphasis has been placed on the need to provide more community-based primary health care services. In areas where these services are not available, families often have to seek attention for health prolems at a local hospital, which is not the ideal place to seek primary health care.

Secondary health care

Secondary health care is provided by more specialised health services. These services include paediatricians (child health specialists), obstetricians (pregnancy and birth specialists), physiotherapists, occupational health therapists, speech pathologists or any one of the many other specialised health services. Outpatient departments at large hospitals provide secondary health care, though recently this is less the case except for chronic health problems. These specialised services are also provided at community health centres and increasingly through private practice.

Tertiary health care

Hospitals are the major providers of tertiary health care. Persons are usually admitted to hospital for treatment and/or surgery. Hospital care can be traumatic to the person and is very expensive to provide. The aim of primary and secondary health care is to prevent and treat illness outside of the hospital environment, thus reducing the need for and cost of tertiary health care. Of all the money allocated to health services in Australia, most goes to hospitals.

It can be argued that if more funds were given to primary health care there would be less pressure on hospitals. An example of this is the current need for hospitals to treat serious conditions such as accidents or heart attacks. Primary health advocates argue that more health education on how to prevent accidents (especially motor vehicle accidents) and how to prevent heart disease would lessen the number of people requiring hospitalisation. This would certainly be best for individuals and the community.

Models of health care

There has been much discussion recently about the 'medical' and 'social' models of health care. Those people who believe only in the social model think that social factors are ignored by many health professionals. Others may think that it is the technological advances of medicine that have helped improve the health of the population and that these advances should not be ignored.

Both groups are correct. Social factors are extremely important to health. There is much evidence that people living in poverty or social isolation have very poor health. Yet nobody would wish to deny these people medical treatment for their ill health. Social justice requires that poverty and social isolation be relieved. Such relief will, in the long term, help to prevent illness, but medical treatment should remain available.

Katya and Jon live with their three young children (all under 5 years of age) in a small 2-bedroom flat in an inner-city area. Jon has been unable to work for several years due to bronchitis and asthma. Katya has a part-time job in a sandwich bar. They receive rent allowance and sickness benefits but find it difficult to make the money last until their next payment comes. This means that the children don't get enough fruit and vegetables for much of the time.

Katya is part of a large extended family and she often looks after her sister's three young children. This means that the flat is very crowded and the children often have colds and runny noses. Sometimes they have middle-ear infections that need treatment. Jon started smoking when he was a teenager. All his mates smoked and he has found it difficult to give it up. He worries that the money he spends on smokes means that his family has less. He knows that his bronchitis, and probably his asthma, is due to his smoking. He goes to the doctor every couple of weeks and is frequently treated for both the asthma and bronchitis.

This family's social situation certainly contributes to their poor health. When Katya has her sister's children in the flat it is very overcrowded. The large number of children under 5 years of age means that it is easy for infection to spread between the children.

The lack of fruit and vegetables for the children means that they are probably not getting adequate nutrients. This causes their general health to be poorer than it should be, which will make it harder for their bodies to resist infection. Poor nutrition in childhood also has a harmful effect on health in adult life.

The children also suffer the consequences of passive smoking. Children who live in a house where someone smokes are more likely to have respiratory infections (National Health and Medical Research Council 1997).

Jon's health suffers from his smoking, which in turn prevents him from working. The worry about this probably makes him smoke more. The whole family suffers from not having enough money.

Ideally, Jon would be helped to give up smoking and get well enough to work. The family would move to a house where there was room for all the children. There would be enough money to enable the family to manage from week to week.

Health professionals should certainly be working with the family and encouraging this to happen. Yet this will take some time, and in the meantime treatment is still needed by the children for their infections and by Jon for his bronchitis and asthma. At the moment this family needs both the social and medical models of health care.

Jon and Katya should not be blamed for their poor health. This would be seen as blaming the victims of social, educational and economic disadvantage.

History of child health in Australia

Health and Australian society

An understanding of the historical aspects of health will help put the current health needs of children in context.

In the past, the major health emphasis was on the prevention and treatment of infectious diseases, which caused most of the deaths and serious illnesses in children.

Improvement in living standards

Improved personal hygiene practices and nutrition during the 20th century has helped to reduce the incidence of many infectious diseases. These social changes, together with the availability of immunisation against major infectious diseases and the introduction of antibiotics, led to an enormous reduction in the mortality (death) rate of infants and young children. The morbidity (sickness) rate also fell. So fewer infants and children were dying or getting sick.

The introduction of community-based maternal and infant health centres to Australia began in the 1930s and they were (and still are) very important in supporting family health. The emphasis is on prevention, and in many places these child or baby health services are known as 'well baby clinics'. Child health is promoted by assessing the growth and development of infants and young children. Any potential health problems can be identified before they become serious. These services can also provide immunisation programs for the prevention of infectious diseases.

This combination of medical and social factors in improving child health is still important today. Children may not be so obviously at risk of the infectious diseases that once caused mortality and morbidity rates in infants and young children to be so high, but the dangers of these diseases returning, and of other diseases appearing, is ever present. It is therefore important that medical and social factors be considered together.

Contemporary community health

Healthy children go together with healthy communities and there are many wider public and community health issues that are important in keeping the population healthy. Australia generally has well developed public health policies and practices.

Traditional public health issues

One of the first responsibilities of public health authorities is to ensure that all water supplies are safe to drink and that sanitation facilities such as sewerage are provided in order to prevent disease. Most Australians have a safe water supply and adequate sanitation, although Aboriginal people living in remote communities, and homeless persons, do not always have access to these services and thus may have a generally poor standard of health.

Immunisation programs are also part of the public health program and are provided free of charge by government agencies in each State and Territory throughout Australia.

Environmental issues

Environmental hazards are becoming an increasing public health issue and the community is rightly concerned about their monitoring and control. These hazards include air quality, radiation, chemicals and food.

An example of what can happen when this monitoring fails is the epidemic of food poisoning that caused both death and serious illness to children in South Australia in 1995. Another example, though fortunately no one died, was the contamination of Sydney's water supply in 1998.

Health education and health promotion

Many programs address problems that come with our lifestyle and our environment. Sun protection practices needed to reduce the high rates of skin cancer have now become part of our culture as 'Slip, Slop, Slap'.

Anti-smoking programs are developed to try to discourage teenagers (or even younger children) from starting to smoke, while programs for adults are aimed at helping them quit.

Other education programs help the community to become more aware of the many diseases related to lifestyle (heart disease, stroke, cancer).

Screening

Screening is another public health measure that is used to detect unsuspected conditions at an early stage and help prevent or treat disease. For example, all babies born in Australian hospitals are screened for a genetic disease called phenylketonuria (PKU), cystic fibrosis and thyroid disease. These conditions are discussed in more detail in Chapter 3.

Pap smears and mammography, which assist in the early recognition of cancer of the cervix and breast, are examples of public health screening for women. Early detection of these forms of cancer leads to treatment before the disease progresses.

Health surveillance

Health surveillance at community-based maternal and child health centres is available for infants and young children. This surveillance charts growth and development so that a failure to grow, any developmental delay or untoward changes are immediately noted and investigated.

Social change and child care

Australian society has seen much social change over the last 20–30 years. This change includes family living and working patterns.

Before the mid 1960s, women generally only worked outside the home if they were very highly qualified professional women who could afford child care in their home or, at the other end of the scale, were very poor and needed to work to survive. Private nannies worked with children of well-off families. Day nurseries and some kindergartens were run by government-sponsored and charitable institutions for children of families in social and economic need.

The women's liberation movement, together with reliable contraception in the form of oral contraceptives, has changed the expectations and opportunities of women in society. Girls stay at school longer and anticipate being able to combine both career and family. Men are no longer the sole wage earners and are expected to share both domestic and child-rearing responsibilities. Many men have found it difficult to adjust to this change and in many families the women have double responsibilities of working both inside and outside the family.

Private child care such as having a nanny in the home has become less affordable, yet the need for child care has grown as more and more women return to work or study for longer periods. A radical change to divorce laws in Australia in the early 1970s has meant that unhappy couples are no longer forced to stay together, and this has brought about a change in social attitude to divorce. It also has resulted in an increasing number of sole-parent families where the caregiving parent needs to work.

A woman's right to work and to have an education has combined with political pressure on governments in Australia to provide child care for those families who need these services. Professional experts in child care and early childhood education, as well as parents, have emphasised the need to ensure that education and care are provided and that child-care facilities are not just 'child minding' centres.

The old-style day nurseries thus have become the child-care centres of today, and the training of staff has changed accordingly. In the past the day nurseries were staffed by registered nurses together with mothercraft nurses. Neither type of nurse had any special training in early childhood education and most had trained in a residential institution. There was much emphasis on health, hygiene and rigid routines, and less on learning activities.

With the new child-care centres has come the demand for staff whose training has a greater emphasis on early childhood education. Thus the mothercraft nurse has given way to the graduate in child-care studies. Bridging courses were put in place for mothercraft nurses. Early childhood teachers also work in child-care centres as well as in the formal education system.

A recent international review of day care for children under school age has shown long-term effects to be positive. This is especially noticeable in children coming from homes in the lower socioeconomic groups of society. The children who had attended day care as young children increased their chances of employment, got better jobs and were less likely to become pregnant as teenagers (Zoritch et al. 1999).

In contemporary Australian society many pre-school-aged children, from a few weeks old to 5 or 6 years of age, now spend many of their waking hours in some form of non-parental child care, whether it be centre-based care, family day care or private care by family or friends. Older children may attend out-of-school-hours programs and vacation programs. The Department of Family and Community Service census of 1999 shows that over 520,000 Australian children attend some type of formal child care.

The social benefits of attending child care have been seen. There are, however, some health concerns we need to note. A large number of babies and young children attend long-day care centres for many hours a day. The grouping together of so many young children has caused infection rates to rise. It may be that some of the health messages from the past have been lost or are forgotten. We do not need to return to the rigid routines of the past. Health routines in contemporary child care can become part of the vibrant learning experiences of the children.

Child health at the beginning of the 21st century

Children who are born in Australia can generally look forward to a long life because the rates of death and serious illnesses amongst infants and young children are low. The standard of living is high, so that many diseases are prevented. Family planning is available, so that families can choose when to have children in order to give them a healthy start to life.

Yet there are still many threats to the health of infants and children and there are many inequalities in health.

Accidents in childhood

A baby in the first year of life faces the hazards of birth and the risk of Sudden Infant Death Syndrome (cot death). Once these hazards are survived, the most likely cause of death or hospitalisation is accidents. Each year too many children die or are hospitalised with serious injuries caused by accidents. This is discussed in detail in Chapter 8.

Nutrition

Australia produces plenty of the nutritious food that is needed to promote and maintain the health of both children and adults. Yet there is much concern among nutritionists that children are not getting adequate nutrients, or that they are consuming too much sugar and fat. The consequences of poor nutrition are life-long and lead to heart disease and perhaps cancer in later life.

Inadequate maternal nutrition leads to babies with low birthweight even at full term. This is of particular concern in developing countries. The long-term consequences of low birthweight are not fully known but there is increasing evidence that it may cause heart disease in young adults (Barker 1994). Nutrition is the topic of Chapter 7.

Social, economic and educational disadvantage

Many of the inequalities in health in Australia are linked to the level of education and economic status (Mathers 1995). Lack of education means adults are less likely to have a well paid job, which then puts them and their family at an economic disadvantage.

Children who live in economically disadvantaged families have been identified by the Australian Health Ministers' Advisory Council (1995) as belonging to one of the groups who are at risk of poor health.

Single-parent families are often economically disadvantaged and have inadequate housing, which can contribute to poor social, emotional and physical health. Those children living in families where one or both parents are unemployed are also at a disadvantage because of poverty.

Single teenage parents are likely to be a special concern, as they are taking responsibility for a baby at a time when most teenagers are still at school completing their secondary education. Teenage mothers may be unable to work due to incomplete education and lack of qualifications. This means that they are likely to live in poverty, which is one of the causes of poor child health.

Refugees and others who have recently arrived in Australia are also at risk of poor health due to both poverty and to the persecution that caused them to become refugees. Many refugees have had very traumatic experiences in the past, involving physical danger, cultural rejection and quite horrific social and emotional stresses.

Emotional and psychological health

During the last three decades of the 20th century the rate of educational, social and emotional problems rose (Williams 1992). This also includes an increase in cases of child abuse: physical, emotional and sexual, as well as basic neglect. The families of these children need support in order to prevent abuse occurring. Censure after the event does not help the abused child.

A study carried out at the TVW Telethon Institute for Child Health Research noted that there were many children who had mental and psychological problems (ABS 1996). Sadly, Australia has the highest adolescent suicide rate of all developed countries (Australian Health Ministers' Advisory Council 1995).

Children with disabilities and chronic illness

A disability is not an illness, but a disabled child will have special health needs, as does a child with a chronic (long-term) illness. Meeting the physical needs of these children has become a real possibility with technological advances such as electric wheel chairs for mobility and computers for communication.

Community attitudes toward children with disabilities are now more positive and accepting than in the past. A lack of socialisation was often a cause for concern before integration of these children into child care and schools became both policy and practice. Support for the family has improved through government support and parent self-help groups.

Child-care centres

Spending time in child care has many educational and social advantages for children. It can, however, also be a potential threat to health, especially in the first 2 years of life. Wherever there are lots of young children, there are lots of germs. Young children are unable to fight these germs as well as older children or adults. So children under two years of age who attend long-day care have many more episodes of infection than do those children in family day care or at home (Skull 1998).

A study carried out in 10 Darwin child-care centres in 1997 showed in any given fortnight of the study:

- 1 in 4 children was taken to a doctor because they were ill;
- 1 in 5 children was sick enough to be kept home from child care;
- 1 in 6 parents had to take time off work;
- 1 in 6 children was prescribed antibiotics for infection. (Skull 1998)

This means that a lot of children are becoming sick because they attend child-care centres. The prevention of infection in child care is examined in Chapters 5 and 6. Any sickness disrupts the social and emotional health of the child and may have negative effects on development and learning.

Current staff-to-child ratios in the under-2-years-old group can make it difficult to quickly meet all the children's many needs at any one time. In *Children First* Penelope Leach (1994) argues that this is because of the immediacy of care needed at this age.

Leonora is working with three babies aged 7, 12 and 14 months in a room that is just off the toddlers' area. The child-staff ratio in her State is 1 : 5 for the under-2-years-old group. She has had a busy morning and one of the staff members from the toddlers' room has come in and helped when things were particularly hectic. Everything is peaceful now. The baby of 12 months is sleeping in his cot at the far end of the room, the 14-month child is pulling himself up and walking between the furniture and Leonora is giving the baby of 7 months a bottle. She does find it difficult to give the baby her full attention and still observe and interact with the toddler, but is just about managing to do this.

Suddenly there is a scream as the toddler falls over. He has slipped and hit his head on a chair as he fell. The baby who has been sleeping wakes with the noise and starts crying with fright. The youngest baby is still trying to feed.

So what does Leonora do? All three children need her immediate attention. In order to assess if the fallen child has injured himself and to comfort him, she needs to interrupt the feeding baby and leave the crying baby alone in his cot. The staff member from the toddlers' room might come in and help again but this means that the toddlers' lunchtime would be interrupted. The director of the centre may well come and assist, but until extra assistance arrives none of these three babies can have their needs met.

Having more staff than is needed to satisfy the regulations would be one solution but this makes child care very expensive. Many parents find it difficult to pay the fees at the current rate.

Leonora knows how important it is for child health to support the babies in all areas of development and worries that sometimes this is very difficult to achieve, even when she has only three babies in her care.

Aboriginal and Torres Strait Islander child health

Cultural alienation

The history of Aboriginal and Torres Strait Islander people since European settlement has been one of alienation from the dominant culture.

It was earlier Government policy to assimilate Aboriginal and Torres Strait Islander people into mainstream society which, until the mid-1940s, was mainly white and English-speaking.

Until 1967, Aboriginal people were not counted in the census as part of the population. They did not have the right to vote or have any of the rights of Australian citizens. In the first half of the twentieth century children who had a non-Aboriginal parent were often forcibly taken away from their families and placed in children's homes or fostered with white families. Many of these children were unaware of their Aboriginality or that they had families living in other parts of Australia. This practice continued to some extent into the 1970s. Many 'stolen children' never knew their family and lived in institutions where they were not in an emotionally close relationship with a caregiver. Many of these people have grown up to become parents and grandparents of city- and town-dwelling Aboriginal children in the current generation.

Aboriginal and Torres Strait Islander people in the past depended on their families and their culture. The weakening of links with traditional family life and culture has had a major impact on the health of many of these people.

Current health status of Aboriginal people

An enormous difference in health status still exists between our indigenous Aboriginal and Torres Strait Islander children and other Australian children. The poor health of indigenous children can create many problems in development, learning and education.

Child care and education should be an agent for social change and health improvement. This is a slow process and one that non-Aboriginal Australians perhaps do not fully understand. Until recently, the full extent of the poor health of Aboriginal and Torres Strait Islander infants and children was not openly acknowledged.

Infant mortality

The death rate for Aboriginal babies was reduced in the last decade of the 20th century, but it is still more than three times that of non-Aboriginal babies.

Infections

Childhood infections among Aboriginal and Torres Strait Islander children are very common, causing the child to be unwell and miss child care or school. In addition, many childhood infections cause serious health complications in later life. Improving the health of Aboriginal children not only has an immediate positive effect on learning, but should enhance health in the long term.

Common infections are:

- Scabies caused by mites which burrow under the skin leading to secondary infection.
- Impetigo (school sores) caused by bacteria that enter through the broken skin of scabies infections. Impetigo, if untreated, may lead to kidney disease and can also contribute to rheumatic fever.
- Gastrointestinal infections, caused both by viruses and bacteria, which cause diarrhoea, weight loss and poor growth.
- Respiratory tract infections caused by viruses and bacteria and which can lead to otitis media (middle-ear infection), bronchitis, pneumonia and sometimes lasting lung damage.
- Parasitic infections, such as intestinal worms, leading to anaemia and malnutrition.

Many of these infections would be prevented if living conditions and hygiene practices were improved. Health education is a vital component of activities in an Aboriginal child-care setting and school and can be integrated into other learning activities.

Links with the local Health Centre staff could lead to better health practices being introduced into child-care settings and schools.

Otitis media (middle-ear infection)

This infection is particularly prevalent among many Aboriginal babies and young children. The condition is described in detail in Chapter 5.

Otitis media causes impaired hearing throughout infancy and early childhood, with consequent negative effects on social and language development and learning. Child-care professionals working with these children really need to have special training in working with children whose hearing is impaired.

Nutrition

The child malnutrition rate in many Aboriginal communities is worse than some countries in Africa. In some Aboriginal communities in the Northern Territory, 25 percent of children under 5 years of age meet the World Health Organization definition of malnutrition (Ruben & Walker 1995). Poor nutrition, like other health problems, not only affects the child at the time but can also lead to poor health in later life.

The diet of Aboriginal people has changed since non-Aboriginal settlers interrupted the traditional lifestyle of hunter-gatherers. Previously the diet of Aboriginal people consisted of lean meat and high-fibre fruit and roots.

Aboriginal people working on pastoral and cattle stations were given rations of flour, tea, sugar and occasional meat, thus poor nutritional practices were encouraged by non-Aboriginal employers.

The relocation of Aboriginal people into settled communities is relatively recent in northern Australia. Living in one place means that the supply of roots, berries and animals can soon be exhausted, thus the major source of food in most communities is the store, which generally stocks poor-quality food at an expensive price. There is no doubt that improving the store food would upgrade the nutritional status of Aboriginal people.

Child-care professionals and teachers have a marvellous opportunity to provide practical nutrition education in Aboriginal child-care settings and schools. This can include gathering food in a traditional way (if possible), growing food, cooking food as well as eating it, and all these activities can enrich many other learning experiences such as science, maths, environmental studies, social and cultural education.

The role of child-care and early-childhood educators in child health

General role

The importance of those working with babies and young children cannot be over-emphasised. Child-care professionals have the responsibility of providing a safe (yet stimulating) environment where the child's nutritional needs are met and where the child's health is maintained. Staff are also expected to recognise the signs of illness in a child and to take appropriate measures in each individual situation.

Health education

Health education for the child also takes place within a child-care setting. Daily routines such as nappy changing, hand washing, dressing and meals provide many opportunities for learning experiences that deliver health education messages. These health messages are for life. A child learns so very much in the first 5 years that is retained throughout life.

Families and health resources

Child-care and early-childhood education professionals are the persons with whom families most frequently communicate about the care and health of their children. There is daily dialogue between staff and parents about what has been happening with the child at the centre and in the home situation.

This dialogue provides an important opportunity for discussion with the parents about health matters. Resources in the form of leaflets that give information about local health facilities, child development, immunisation programs, child safety, nutrition and other related issues should also be available for parents.

Other health professionals

Child-care and early-childhood educators are an important part of community health services. Children and families are best supported when all services are integrated and cooperation exists between staff. This is done on a formal basis in some places where the child and family health clinic, pre-school, child-care centre and family day care coordinators are situated in the one centre.

Informal arrangements to link services may be made in other places. Sometimes it is hard for families to get the support they need because child health, education and family services are all in different government departments (see Chapter 12).

Families and child care

Child-care facilities play a very important role in promoting the all-round health of the family. 'Child care' should perhaps be more correctly named 'family care', as the child comes into the children's service as part of a family and brings with him/her a history of past experiences.

Family structures have changed over the last 30 years and, along with the fact that Australian society has become so culturally diverse, there is a wide range of interesting differences within our society. Here are some examples of how child care provides a health service to families.

CASE STUDY 1

Maria and Joe are Australian-born and live with their two children, Angela (3 years) and Peter (9 months), in their own home in an outer suburb of a large city. Both Maria's and Joe's parents were born in Italy but came to Australia as young children and had all their schooling here. Joe is a self-employed carpenter and Maria has recently returned from maternity leave to her clerical position in the public service. Their families knew each other before Maria and Joe married and they see each other often, as well as getting together at weekends, on special occasions and holidays.

Angela and Peter both attend a local day-care centre full time. Their grandparents work part-time and live near enough to sometimes pick up the children from child care. So grandparents, parents and children see each other frequently.

Peter and Angela are living within a nuclear family with their biological parents, yet they have close contact with grandparents and other family members. This family is able to give social and emotional support to each other because they all live nearby, and because some of the old cultural values of Italian families have been maintained. Both Angela's mother and mother-in-law are happy to help care for the children in the evenings and at the weekend and to listen when she has concerns about bringing up a family.

The child-care centre is still an essential part of their lives. Maria and Joe both need to work in order to pay their home mortgage, and all grandparents work part-time. The staff in the child-care centre know all the family members and value the wide social, cultural and emotional experiences that the children share.

CASE STUDY 2

Donna and Ian have been married for 10 years and have moved six times during their married life. Ian, who is in the armed forces, is happy to move, as it nearly always means promotion, and Donna has supported him in this. The moves have taken them to Western Australia, Victoria and far north Queensland. They have three children aged 2, 5 and 8 and

Continued

the family now lives in Darwin, where they have been for 8 months. Donna's parents live in Hobart. Ian's father died a year ago and his mother has recently moved to Melbourne from a country town in Victoria so that she can be near her daughter's family. The high cost of fares to the Northern Territory from the southern States means that it is difficult for the grandparents to visit Darwin.

Donna has tried many times to finish a degree course in education, as she would like to be a teacher when her youngest child has started school. She has found the moving around difficult with her studies as each university has a different course. She is now enrolled part-time and hopes they stay long enough in Darwin for her to complete her course. She has joined classes where the rest of the students have known each other for more than 2 years and has found this to be socially difficult.

Donna needs child care for 2 days a week and after-school care for 2 afternoons each week. She will need full-time care for the 4 weeks she is on teaching practice.

Donna and Ian have lived in many places. At each move Ian has had his work and the social structure this gives him. The armed services do provide family support, housing and other social contacts and these have helped Donna and the children settle into each new place. It has always been her responsibility to sort out her university enrolments and the child care she will need to enable her to get to classes. Ian is totally supportive of her doing the course and certainly helps with housework and child care when he is at home, but his job takes him out bush a lot and at these times Donna is quite alone. In some ways it was easier when she lived on the armed services base, as the other service wives were understanding and they helped each other out. Her accommodation is now within the civilian community in a pleasant house that is rented by the services

Donna is unable to have close contact with her extended family. She can ring her mother but misses just being able to drop round for a cup of tea to discuss family life and any concerns about bringing up her children. Her extended family cannot pick children up after school.

The child-care centre provides Donna with contact with other parents, with staff who know her 2-year-old well and with whom she can share any concerns. The staff are helpful if Donna needs extra hours of care when she has essays due; they are interested in her course and are trying to arrange things for the 4 weeks she will be on practice teaching. The child-care centre is also another link with the civilian population and the activities that are happening around town. After-school care also gives encouragement and the security of knowing her children are busy and happy.

CASE STUDY 3

Jemma is 17 and lives alone in an inner city flat with Dominic, her son, who is 8 months old. She occasionally sees Ernst (19), the baby's father, who sometimes gives her money but Ernst is unemployed and doesn't have much money.

Jemma's parents divorced when she was 4 and she has scarcely seen her father since that time. Her mother lives in the country with her second husband and has three children who are still in primary school. Jemma's mother sends clothes and toys for Dominic whenever she can. They can only get to see each other every 3–4 months.

Dominic is a generally happy baby. He was breast fed until recently and now eats mashed-up food and drinks formula from a bottle. Jemma has taken him regularly to the Community Health Centre and his weight gain and developmental progress are fine. He is fully immunised.

It is lonely through the day, as most of her friends are still at school or at work, and Jemma does not have spare money to go out much. She tends to watch the soaps a fair bit and is beginning to get rather bored. Dominic has begun to crawl, and she knows she will need to clean up the floor so that it is safe for him to get around. Today she got rather cross with him, as he picked up an open brooch she had dropped on the floor. She felt mean, as she knew it was her fault for leaving it around. Soon he will need somewhere to play, and she lives on the 16th floor of the flats.

Jemma wonders what it would be like to go off and do a course and get a job, but worries about who would care for Dominic and how much it would cost.

Jemma is one of the number of teenagers who become sole parents each year. Her contact with the baby's father is irregular and she is unable to see her own mother very often. Not being able to get out much during the day, she is becoming increasingly socially isolated. She has gained support from the Community Health nurses and Dominic is healthy and active, but his surroundings are limited and he will soon start to need more space to explore and in which to play.

Getting a qualification and a job will not only extend Jemma's horizons but will also provide positive experiences for Dominic. Child-care staff will be sensitive to Jemma's needs and discuss with her Dominic's activities during the day. Jemma will get ideas for suitable activities at home and also have access to information on child development and how to cope with different behaviours. Any health and developmental changes or concerns will be immediately noticed. Dominic will have qualified staff caring for him and providing appropriate learning experiences. He will have space to play outside and mix with other children.

Jemma will be eligible for the maximum rate of Child Care Benefit for child care fees. Centrelink staff can also tell her about any training schemes she might join. Gaining a job will increase Jemma's income and widen her social contacts.

Jemma may well meet other parents whose children attend child care or attend her training college, and informal support groups can grow from these meetings.

CASE STUDY 4

Tran is 32 years old and is a refugee from Cambodia. She came to Australia 4 years ago with her husband Mal. She has no idea what has happened to the rest of her family, apart from her father, as they were all sent to different refugee camps in Thailand and other places. She knows her father died of starvation during the Pol Pot regime. Tran and Mal were accepted by Australia as refugees, but not before they had a fearful trip by boat, when they were attacked by pirates and many women were raped. Tran still has dreadful nightmares about this.

Mal, who worked as a business manager in Cambodia, has an unskilled job in a timber yard. He has an easygoing personality, the other employees have accepted him well, and he enjoys the friendliness of his workmates. He knew some English before coming to Australia and has become fairly fluent since starting work. He and Tran speak Cambodian at home and with some of their neighbours.

Tran and Mal live in a rented flat in an area of a city where there are many other refugees, but would like to buy their own house or flat. This has become very important as they now have a baby son (Banth) who is 14 months old. They would like him to grow up having all the educational opportunities that they have now lost and which they value so highly.

Tran has recently completed an English course in the evenings at a local college and is now feeling much more confident about looking for work, which she will need to do in order to save for their own home, as long as she can find child care for Banth.

Tran and Mal have been displaced from their family and culture and suffered many traumatic experiences. They have no extended family, though they are friendly with some of their neighbours who are also refugees. Mal's workmates are friendly but they do not socialise outside of work hours.

Tran is home all day caring for Banth and she enjoys this, although she sometimes feels very lonely. She knows that she will need to work in paid employment if they are to save for a house.

Child care for this family could help with the maintenance of their Cambodian culture while helping the family settle into Australian society.

Many child-care centres employ multilingual staff, especially in areas where there are languages other than English spoken. Banth would be surrounded by both English and Cambodian as he starts to talk. Children who are exposed to more than one language become fluent in each language with no confusion. He would also sing Cambodian songs and chant rhymes and have stories read to him in this language as well as in English.

A strong cultural identity is very important for health, and maintaining Cambodian culture will not diminish Tran, Mal or Banth's commitment to Australian society.

CASE STUDY 5

Selina is an Aboriginal woman who is 20. She and her two children, aged 3 and 4, live with her mother and stepfather in a large country town. Selina doesn't know who her own biological father is and her mother refuses to discuss it. Ted, who is Selina's partner and father of the children, works in another State; he gets home to see everyone as often as he can and sends money regularly.

Both Ted's and Selina's mothers were taken from their families in remote communities when very young and sent to children's homes in a city. Ted's mother ran away when she was 14 and went back to her community, where she found her mother. Ted's mother still lives in the community.

Selina's mother was sent to work as a housemaid in another State and never knew her own mother or where she came from until a year ago. She found her mother had died five years before, but she did meet some aunts and cousins with whom she now keeps in touch.

Continued

Selina doesn't get on too well with her mother and they tend to argue a lot. Her mother wanted her to stay on at school but Selina refused and played truant all the time until she became pregnant. She had been going out with Ted for a couple of months when this happened, so they went off to see Ted's mother and stayed living in the community. This didn't work out as neither of them had jobs and Selina became pregnant again very quickly after the first baby was born. The children were always getting sick, which worried Selina. So when Ted heard of jobs going on a mine in another State, he decided to give it a go and Selina moved back into her mother's house.

The house is very small and Selina and the children have to share a bedroom. Her stepfather gets very cross with the children when they make a noise while he is watching television. Occasionally he hits them very hard. They are both active, restless children and shout a lot.

The children have missed out on health surveillance due to the moves and Selina thinks they may be a bit skinny after being sick so much in the community.

Selina is also restless. She loves Ted and the children but wishes she had taken her mother's advice and stayed at school. It wasn't that she found the work difficult, almost the opposite, but she got bored with it all and felt no one really liked her because she was Aboriginal, though nobody actually said anything directly.

Because Selina's and Ted's mothers are both from the 'stolen generation', they grew up knowing little about their families or their culture. Many of these children also grew up without affection and without forming real attachments, which often causes serious social and emotional deprivation.

Selina has never known about her father and she has only just met some of her mother's aunts and cousins. She is fond of her stepfather but wishes he wouldn't get so impatient with the children, though she knows they make a lot of noise.

Her own relationship with Ted is difficult to maintain, with him working in another State. She is not sure if they are really still partners, and it is difficult to find a private place to talk when he comes to see her and the children.

The town has several child-care centres, including one for staff and students at the local Vocational Education and Training college. The college may have bridging courses that would lead to further education for Selina.

The child-care centre would provide more physical space for the children to engage in energetic activities. Staff at the child-care centre would also notice the loudness and restlessness of Selina's two children and set up some formal observations after discussing this with her. It may be that the illnesses they had while living in the remote community has left them with some hearing impairment due to chronic middle-ear infection.

Hearing tests can be done to assess whether they have any hearing loss, while at the same time assessing the children's general health and growth status. Treatment may be needed if any infection remains. Staff at the child-care centre can arrange the environment and program to help the children communicate more easily and will discuss these measures with Selina, who can also do things at home to help the children. A speech therapist will nearly always be part of the health team assessing and treating the children. Selina's stepfather might well be much more patient knowing that there is a reason why the children have been so noisy.

CASE STUDY 6

Belinda is in her mid-thirties and married to Jim. Both work in medical research at a large city institution. They have one child, Emma, who is 3 months old. Belinda has been on maternity leave but now wishes to return to work. She has a very interesting and challenging research project to complete, but is feeling worried about leaving Emma.

Neither Belinda nor Jim has any relatives in Australia, having come from England to work here after finishing their doctorates. They enjoyed it so much that they took out Australian citizenship and plan to bring up their family here.

Jim and Belinda have had time to look at different child-care options for their family. They have visited several centres but think Emma is still too young to be with so many other children. They have also chatted with the Family Day Care coordinator at the local Council and are pleased with the way the scheme is run and the positive encouragement that is given to caregivers to gain qualifications.

The Family Day Care coordinator set up several visits and interviews with prospective caregivers so Belinda and Jim had a chance to find child care that would be complementary to their way of life. The choice turned out to be easier than expected, as they felt immediately comfortable with the second caregiver they met, and Emma seemed to like her as well.

Continued

There are three other children, aged 2, 3 and 4, attending this family day-care home. All the children have been there since they were a few months old. The caregiver has two children of her own but they are both at school. Belinda and Jim liked the way the caregiver and the children interacted with each other. They were pleased with the number of interesting activities available from which the children could choose. They especially liked the way the caregiver greeted Emma, warmly but without crowding or overwhelming the baby. In response Emma looked and smiled and made lots of gooing noises.

Belinda and Jim are looking for a smaller child-care setting and have chosen family day care, where Emma will be with only three other children during the day. Emma will experience another style of family life with values close to her own, but different enough to provide her with experiences she would not get at home. These experiences may well, in part, compensate for the lack of extended family.

Belinda and Jim will form a positive relationship with the caregiver and chat to her each morning and evening about what has been happening with Emma. There are already signs that Emma will become attached to the caregiver and that there will be cuddles as well as activities throughout the day.

As Emma grows, she will benefit from being with other children, being taken to play group and to pre-school.

Belinda and Ben have busy careers and feel that the home setting of family day care will best suit Emma and their lifestyle.

Children in other countries

Good health is the right of all children though, sadly, not all children in the world are given this right. In many developing countries maternal and infant mortality rates are still unacceptably high. Many babies and young children still die from preventable infectious diseases. For instance, malaria is very prevalent in tropical countries and cerebral malaria kills and disables children. Basic sanitation in many places is non-existent. There is no sewerage or clean water supply. Water from wells is often contaminated and causes fatal diarrhoeal diseases. The food supply is dependent on the weather. A drought or flood causes food to be very scarce, and children starve.

A lack of family planning facilities means that the birth rate remains very high, although it is very hard to care for large families. Medical supplies are often unavailable due to the cost, so treatment is very basic. Many children die from diseases that would be easily treated in Australia.

Most people in these countries are very poor. Schools, when they are available, may not be free. Consequently many children have no education and cannot read or write. Often young children are sent out to work.

The health of the children in these countries could be improved by education. The World Health Organization has identified that the mother's level of education is the single most important factor that leads toward improving the health of children in these countries. This makes education for girls and women a very important issue.

Learning activities

1. What types of child-care services are available in your area—eg: family day care, long-day centre-based care, occasional care, out-of-school-hours care, vacation care?
2. List all the community health services available for families in your area. Collect some information leaflets about what these services provide for your own information and for parents.

References

Australian Bureau of Statistics (1996). *Western Australian child health survey: Family and community well-being in the 1990s*. Canberra, Australian Government Publishing Service (AGPS).

Australian Health Ministers' Advisory Council (1995). *The health of young Australians*. Canberra, AGPS.

Barker DJP. (1994). *Mothers, babies and disease in later life*. London, BMJ Publishing Group.

Leach P. (1994). *Children first*. Harmondsworth, Penguin.

Mathers C. (1998). The health consequences of unemployment: The evidence. *Medical Journal of Australia*, 168(4):178–182.

National Health and Medical Research Council (NHMRC). (1997). *The health effects of passive smoking*. Canberra, AGPS.

Ruben AR, Walker AC. (1995). Malnutrition among rural Aboriginal children in the Top End of the Northern Territory. *Medical Journal of Australia*, 162(8):400–403.

Skull S. (1998). Unpublished MPH thesis, National Centre for Epidemiology and Public Health, Australian National University, Canberra.

Williams H. in Clements A. ed. (1992). *Infant and family health in Australia*. Melbourne, Churchill Livingstone.

World Health Organization (1978). *Declaration of Alma Ata*. International Conference on Primary Health Care. Alma Ata. (The definition was reinforced at this conference).

Zoritch B, Roberts I, Oakley A. (1999). The health and welfare effects of pre-school day care. Day care for pre-school children (Cochrane Review), in *The Cochrane Library*, Issue 3, Update Software.

Further reading

Australian Institute of Health and Welfare (AIHW) (2000). *Australia's health 2000: The seventh biennial health report of the Australian Institute of Health and Welfare*. Canberra, AIHW.

Fahey K. (1995). Poverty, welfare and single mothers: A primary health concern. *Journal of the Australian College of Midwives*, 8(1):18–23.

Garton AF, Zubrick SR, Silburn SR. (1995). The Western Australian child health survey: A pilot study. *Australian and New Zealand Journal of Psychiatry*, 29(1):48–57.

Mathews JD. (1997). Historical, social and biological understanding is needed to improve Aboriginal health. *Recent Advances in Microbiology*, Vol 15, 257–334.

Reid J, Trompf P, eds. (1990). *The health of immigrant Australia*. Sydney, Harcourt, Brace, Jovanovich.

Reid J, Trompf P, eds. (1991). *The health of Aboriginal Australia*. Sydney, Harcourt, Brace, Jovanovich.

Ochiltree G. (1990). *Children in Australian families*. Melbourne, Longman Cheshire.

Ochiltree G. (1994). *Effects of child care on young children*. Melbourne, Australian Institute of Family Studies.

Weeks W, Wilson J, eds. (1995). *Issues facing Australian families*. Melbourne, Longman.

CHAPTER 2

Choosing to have children

ALL CHILDREN SHOULD be wanted children. This is a basic principle of child health and wellbeing. Children who are wanted are more likely to be healthy and have the best care and education opportunities. Their families are well prepared for the pregnancy, the birth and the demands of child rearing. For most Australians it is possible, and usually necessary too, to plan families, to choose when to have children.

In the past, when contraception was generally unreliable, families were much larger and the numbers of child deaths and illness were much greater than it is now.

Most women and couples in contemporary Australia use some form of contraception (birth control/family planning) at some time in their reproductive lives. Different forms of contraception suit different people, different lifestyles and different stages of life. Religious and cultural values also play an important part in decisions about contraception and family size.

It is not the role of child-care and early childhood education professionals to give contraceptive advice, but information about where such advice can be obtained should be available for parents and for staff members too.

Information about disease prevention should also be available for staff and parents. This includes information regarding safe sex practices. The danger of sexual transmission of HIV (Human Immunodeficiency Virus) which leads to AIDS (Acquired Immune Deficiency Syndrome), or Hepatitis B and C and other diseases must not be underestimated.

Conception (fertilisation) and contraception

Conception or fertilisation is when the male spermatozoa enters the female egg (ovum) of the woman, thus causing an embryo to start developing. Contraception is the prevention of this conception or fertilisation.

Human reproductive systems

An understanding of the human reproductive systems is useful when looking at how contraception works. Terms that are often used relating to body systems are:

- Anatomy, or structure: What the body is made up of—tissues, bones and organs.
- Physiology, or function: How all these structures and body parts work.

The female reproductive system

Structure

The female reproductive system (Figure 2.1) is made up of:

- 2 ovaries, which are almond-sized organs on each side of the pelvic area
- 2 fallopian tubes
- The uterus and its different parts:
    - fundus or top
    - body or middle
    - cervix or neck
    - endometrium or lining
- Vagina

Function

The ovaries produce eggs (ova). All the ova are in place in the ovary when a female child is born and, once adolescence is reached, one egg (ovum) is ripened and released from one ovary each 28 days or so. This is called ovulation. The ovum goes into the fallopian tube, where it moves slowly toward the uterus waiting to meet sperm from the male. The woman is fertile each month from the time she ovulates until the time the egg reaches the uterus.

Conception (fertilisation) occurs if a sperm cell (one of millions in an ejaculation) enters the ovum. This happens in the fallopian tube, and the fertilised egg begins dividing into many cells as it travels down to the uterus. Here it implants itself in the endometrium (the lining of the

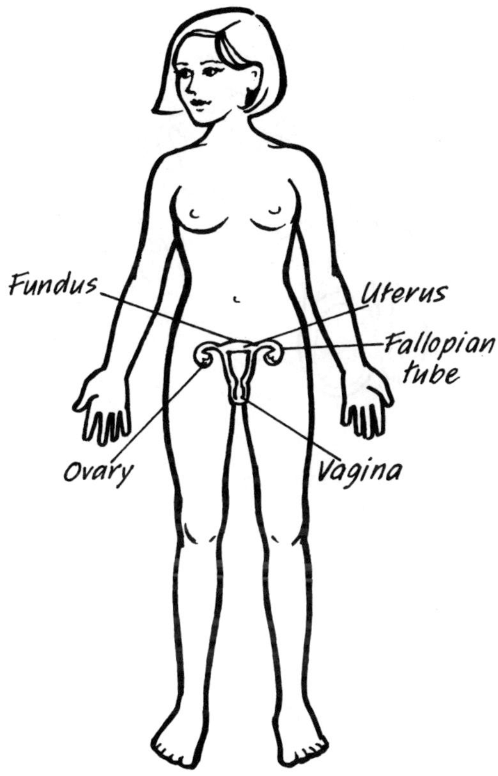

Figure 2.1 Female reproductive system

uterus), which is swollen with blood and other nutrients necessary for the growth of the embryo that develops from the egg after conception.

If fertilisation does not occur, then the egg and the blood-rich endometrium are not needed and are passed out of the body through the vagina as the woman's menstrual period. The menstrual cycle then starts again and occurs about every 28 days, though there are many individual variations as to the time of the cycle.

A woman's fertile life lasts from menarche, which is the time of the first period (usually around 11–14 years of age) until menopause, which is the time of the last period when the woman is around 50 years old.

The male reproductive system

This looks more complicated than that of the female because of the way the tubes loop over each other. Figure 2.2 is a side view of the male reproductive system.

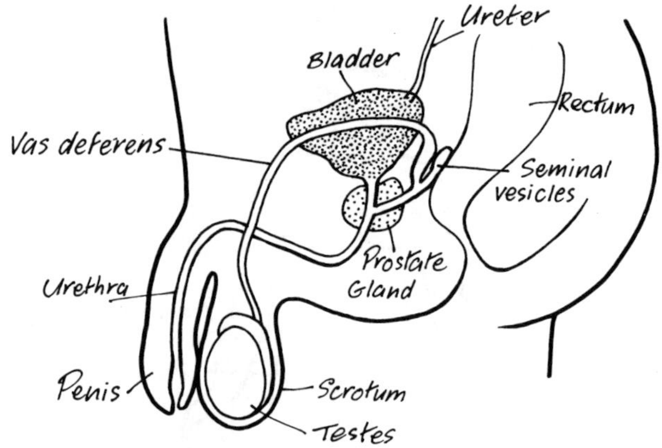

Figure 2.2 Male reproductive system

Structure

The main components are:

- 2 testes found in the scrotum
- 2 vas deferens
- 2 seminal vesicles
- prostate gland
- urethra

Function

Millions of sperm are made in the testes and travel up through the vas deferens to the seminal vesicles. Here they are stored until they are needed during sexual activity and ejaculation.

When the male becomes sexually aroused, fluid from the prostate gland is added to the sperm to form semen. This fluid creates extra pressure as the semen is ejaculated from the body, giving the sperm a 'boost' and thus a better chance of reaching a waiting ovum. The urethra, through which the semen is ejaculated, is also part of the urinary system.

Sperm ejaculated into the woman's vagina goes into the uterus through the cervical opening and then up into the fallopian tubes. Sperm can stay alive in the tubes for several days waiting for an ovum to fertilise.

At adolescence, a boy will have nocturnal emissions of semen (wet dreams) which is an indication of sexual maturity. Unlike women, who reach a definite end to their productive life with menopause, men are fertile all their lives, though they are less fertile as they get older.

Sex hormones

The structure and function of both the male and female reproductive systems is dependent on hormones (chemicals) produced by the pituitary gland in the brain and by the ovaries in the female and the testes in the male. This will be discussed further in Chapter 4.

Contraception

The aim of any contraceptive method is to prevent the sperm from reaching the ovum as it travels down the fallopian tube, remembering that the sperm contains millions of spermatozoa and there is only one ovum. It is as though fate is stacked against the female, though, in evolutionary terms, this has helped to ensure the survival of the human species.

There are many methods of contraception and their reliability often depends on the way they are used.

Abstinence from penetration during sexual activity

This is still the best method of contraception and safe sex. It is, however, sometimes difficult to achieve, as sexual arousal usually leads to a desire for sexual intercourse of the penetrative type. One of the positive aspects of health education in the prevention of HIV/AIDS, Hepatitis B and C and other sexually transmitted diseases is that safe methods of sexual expression other than penetration have been identified and discussed much more openly than has happened in the past.

Barrier methods

These methods physically separate the sperm from the ovum and are available for both males and females.

Condoms

These are latex sheaths that cover the erect penis and are shaped to collect the ejaculated semen at the tip of the condom. As with all other forms of contraception, condoms need to be used correctly and are best used in conjunction with a spermicide, when they give almost 100 percent protection. The condom needs to be gently rolled onto an erect penis, watching out for jagged fingernails. Room should be left at the tip for the ejaculate. A water-based lubricant can be used if needed. The male should hold the bottom of the condom onto the base of his penis as soon as ejaculation occurs, and withdraw the condom and penis from the woman's vagina. This prevents semen from seeping round the base of the condom and into the vagina as the male erection subsides after ejaculation.

Condoms have many advantages, the main one being that they also prevent the spread of sexually transmitted diseases. Other advantages are that they are relatively inexpensive, easily available and need only be used when protection is needed. For these reasons condoms are used by many young people who may or may not be in a long-term relationship. Females, as well as males, should be encouraged to carry some when sexual activity is a possibility.

Using condoms can become part of the sexual foreplay of a couple during arousal. This then prevents condoms being forgotten. It is all too easy for a young couple, say after a party and a few drinks, to be overcome by sexual arousal which causes them to forget to use a condom or to mistakenly think in all the excitement that having sex once without protection will not matter. The power of passion often causes the demise of rational behaviour! Many pregnancies have thus occurred, as well as the contracting of sexually transmitted diseases.

Care should be taken when storing condoms, as the latex does not last in hot conditions such as the glove box of a car or in hip pockets.

Thought should also be given to the safe disposal of used condoms as they may contain infectious material and, in any case, are aesthetically displeasing to other people.

Female condoms, which form a barrier lining within the vagina, are becoming more easily available though they are still not widely used.

Diaphragms or cervical caps

These are caps of a rubber material which cover the top of the vagina or the cervix of the uterus to prevent sperm from getting into the uterus and then up into the fallopian tubes.

Diaphragms and caps need to be the correct size. Women are not all the same measurements inside, just as they are not on the outside. This usually means a visit to a medical practitioner or family planning clinic to be fitted and to learn how to put them in and how to remove them correctly. Caps and diaphragms must also be used with a spermicide as an added precaution.

It is important that diaphragms and caps are put in before sexual intercourse and that they are left in place for 6–8 hours after ejaculation has occurred. This is because the sperm remains active in the vagina for some time after sexual activity.

Caps and diaphragms have been used successfully by many women, but the main risk is that they may not be inserted correctly, which allows sperm to get into the upper part of the vagina and then into the uterus and fallopian tube. Another cause of failure is removing the diaphragm too soon. Caps and diaphragms do not give protection against sexually transmitted diseases.

Unlike condoms, caps and diaphragms can be used many times. They need to be washed after each use, and checked for holes. They should also be stored in a safe place to prevent them being damaged. Women who leave caps and diaphragms in an accessible place in the bathroom sometimes find them being used as bathtime toys by their young children!

Couples in long-term relationships who already have one or more children often choose this method of contraception while they decide if they wish to have more children. More young women are also using diaphragms successfully.

Spermicides (substances that kill sperm)

There are many types of spermicides such as foams, tablets, suppositories and creams. They can be purchased easily at a chemist but are not contraceptives if used alone. They should be used in conjunction with a barrier method such as condom, cap or diaphragm in order to give an extra degree of protection.

Spermicides should be inserted into the vagina, using the correct applicator, immediately prior to sexual intercourse, as the spermicide melts away quite quickly.

Hormonal contraception

Oral contraceptives

Oral contraceptive pills alter the hormonal balance of the menstrual cycle so that ovulation does not occur. Thus there is no ovum for the sperm to fertilise.

Australian women were enthusiastic users of oral contraceptives when they were first available in the early 1960s. These initial pills had a fairly high hormone level and were found to have side effects of weight gain, nausea and headaches in the short term. In the long term, there were heightened risks of blood clots that caused strokes. These risks were quite low if the woman was a non-smoker. It should be remembered that at no time has taking oral contraceptives been as risky as the potential complications of pregnancy.

Oral contraceptives now contain a much lower dose of hormones and still give contraceptive protection. These pills should be taken at the same time every day, and human error in forgetting to take the pill is the main cause of failure.

Correctly used oral contraceptives have a very high rate of success. The main disadvantages are that a doctor's prescription is needed, with follow-up visits to check on the woman's health. Remembering to regularly take the pill each day causes problems for some women. It is important if there are young children in the house that the pills are kept safely out of reach, and this measure in itself causes women to forget to take the pill each day.

Young couples who wish to have children at a later stage might choose this method.

Injectable contraceptives

A progesterone compound is the most common injectable hormone given for contraception. It has the advantage that it only needs to be given every three months.

There is still some debate as to whether this injection should be used on a regular basis for contraceptive purposes, as it was initially developed as a treatment for ovarian cancer. Women using this type of contraceptive often cease to menstruate while they are using the drug. It is, however, becoming more widely used by Australian women for contraceptive purposes and is sometimes recommended by Family Planning Association clinics. It can be useful for women with heavy periods who do not have an increased risk of breast cancer for any other reason.

Hormonal implants

These implants are inserted under the skin of the woman and will give protection against pregnancy for 3 years. A new implant is inserted after this time. Advice from the Family Planning Association or a medical practitioner is needed before this type of device can be made available.

Male contraceptive pill

Much research has been going on to find a hormone that will stop men from producing sperm and it is expected that such a pill will soon be available. Trials are now underway in Britain, South Africa and China and the early results are very promising.

Intrauterine devices (IUDs)

These devices have been used by some cultures in various forms throughout history. It is thought that Arabic people, in past times, used to put stones into the uterus of a camel in order to prevent the camel becoming pregnant. Grafenberg rings, which are an earlier larger version of the smaller IUDs used now, were used by many women in the early 20th century.

Intrauterine devices are inserted through the vagina and cervical opening into the uterus. The insertion must be carried out by a trained person. A 'string' is left hanging through the cervix into the vagina and this is used to check that the IUD is in place. It is recommended that women check that they can feel the tag each month at least, usually after a menstrual period, to ensure that the device is still in place.

The way that IUDs prevent pregnancy is not totally certain. One suggestion is that the ovum, instead of wandering slowly down the fallopian tube, moves much more quickly thus preventing fertilisation occurring. Another suggestion is that fertilisation might occur but that the fertilised ovum cannot implant in the endometrium due to the IUD being in the uterus.

There is a high success rate in preventing pregnancy using IUDs. The advantages are that the contraceptive cover is continuous and that the woman does not have to remember to take a pill or to insert a diaphragm or cap, nor does either partner need to remember to purchase condoms. The IUD is often used as a contraceptive method in between children. It has been successfully used by many women in developing countries.

The disadvantages are that IUDs do not prevent STDs and some women have heavy and painful periods. There is also the risk, albeit very slight, of infection that can travel up the tubes, blocking them and causing permanent sterility. For this reason IUDs are only recommended for women in long-term, stable monogamous relationships.

Sterilisation

It is important that there is adequate preparation and thought before sterilisation of either male or female is performed. It should be seen as permanent, even though some people have had it reversed with the use of microsurgery. This is a costly procedure.

The social and ethical difficulties arising from sterilisation are, in the main, due to social change. A couple may have two or three children, which is their chosen number, and then decide that one partner will be sterilised to prevent any unplanned pregnancy. The relationship may break up some time later and the sterilised person may get a new partner with whom he/she would like to have children. This is an all-too-frequent ethical dilemma these days when health funds are limited: does the community spend money on the very natural desire for a couple to have children when one of the partners has voluntarily in the past chosen to be sterilised?

Female sterilisation

In this procedure the fallopian tubes of the woman are surgically blocked so that any ovum leaving the ovaries cannot get down the tube, and sperm cannot get up to meet the ovum. Fertilisation can therefore not occur. Ova are still released from the ovaries each month and are absorbed into the general abdominal contents. The sterilised woman will still have periods, as there is no interference with any of the hormonal functions of the body.

As this is a surgical procedure, women need to attend a hospital. They may only need to be a day patient, though some women still stay in overnight as a general anaesthetic is needed.

The procedure is performed using a laparoscope, which is a long tube with a light and instruments on the end of it. The surgeon inserts the laparoscope through the abdominal wall, usually under the umbilicus, and then finds the two fallopian tubes and blocks each one off using special clips.

Male sterilisation

This procedure does not usually require hospitalisation and is mostly carried out under local anaesthetic. The surgeon finds the two vas deferens and cuts and ties each off so that sperm from the testes cannot get up to the seminal vesicles to be ejaculated into the woman. This is known as a vasectomy.

It needs to be remembered that the seminal vesicles store sperm, so the male is not immediately sterile after the vasectomy but needs to have sperm specimens analysed for 3 to 4 weeks afterwards until the sperm count is zero.

Some men have been reluctant to have a vasectomy because of the concern that they will not be able ejaculate, which is an essential part of a male orgasm. It is only the sperm that are blocked off, not the fluid in which they were once carried, so a male after vasectomy ejaculates fluid which is made in the prostate gland and which does not contain any sperm. Thus the man loses no sexual feelings nor the ability to ejaculate.

Natural methods

There are several methods of contraception (usually called birth control) that do not use barriers or hormones or any other method that interferes in any way with the functioning of the normal reproductive systems. These methods are approved of by religious persons and institutions such as the Catholic church who do not officially approve of other methods.

Rhythm method

In the past, couples have needed to have a rough guess as to when ovulation might be occurring and to abstain from sex during these estimated times. This was known as the rhythm method, which might have been safe if the woman had a very regular menstrual cycle. The rhythm method proved very unreliable for women who were irregular, or during times such as breastfeeding or early menopause.

It is now easier to recognise with more accuracy when the woman may be ovulating. There are two main ways of doing this:

Temperature check: A woman's basal (lowest) body temperature rises very slightly around the time she ovulates. The basal temperature needs to be measured before rising in the morning while the woman is still at rest. The temperature change is only around a few points of a degree centigrade, so the thermometer used and the method of taking should be the same every day to obtain the most accurate reading. Ideally women should take their basal temperature daily over several menstrual cycles in order to accurately assess when they ovulate. Sexual intercourse should be avoided for several days before the expected ovulation time, during the identified time and for several days afterwards.

Again, this method suits women with regular menstrual cycles. Inaccuracies occur when a woman has an infection or some other condition that may alter her basal temperature.

Cervical mucus (Billings method): Mucus is secreted from the cervix throughout the menstrual cycle. At the time of ovulation there is a change in the chemical structure (pH) of the mucus. Women can recognise the change in their cervical discharge or use a specially prepared piece of paper to test their cervical discharge and accurately recognise the time of ovulation. Sexual intercourse should be avoided during this time.

Two Melbourne medical practitioners (Billings 1983) have developed this method, which has been successful for many couples. These couples are often those in long-term stable relationships where religious beliefs prevent the use of other forms of contraception and where both partners wish to be responsible for birth control.

'Methods' to avoid

There are two 'methods' which are unreliable and should not be used.

Withdrawal

The formal name for withdrawal is *coitus interruptus* and is described in the Bible as the man spilling his seed onto the ground. It has therefore been around a long time. This method relies on the man withdrawing his penis from the woman's vagina before he begins to ejaculate. There are two main problems to this. The first is that some semen is secreted when the man is first sexually aroused, in order to lubricate the tip of the penis, and even this small amount of semen may contain millions of spermatozoa. The second problem is that it is often difficult for the man to tell exactly when he is going to ejaculate and he may pull out too late.

Vaginal douching

This is another very old-fashioned method which involves the woman washing out her vagina immediately after intercourse. Douching does not prevent pregnancy, does not protect against sexually transmitted diseases and is potentially dangerous.

Abortion

Abortion is the medical term for any pregnancy that ends before the baby is viable. A spontaneous abortion is usually called a miscarriage and occurs for many reasons, most of which cannot be identified. An induced abortion is where the pregnancy is terminated intentionally.

Induced abortion

This is not a method of contraception but rather the removal of the embryo or fetus after pregnancy has been established. This method is still not formally legal in Australia, although it is safely obtainable through referral within the health system. Most medical practitioners who are prepared to carry out abortions would prefer to do the procedure before the woman is 12 weeks pregnant as this is thought to be not only physically safest but also less psychologically traumatic. From a legal point of view the principle is to allow abortions when the risk of pregnancy to the woman in health, social and other terms is thought to be significant.

Induced abortion often raises many ethical issues relating to personal values and religious beliefs and there is sometimes public debate about these values and beliefs. Many of those against abortion feel that it is always wrong.

Some persons think abortion should only be done in exceptional circumstances, such as in cases of rape or where there is a known serious malformation of the embryo. Other people think the decision relating to abortion should be only that of the woman and/or the couple.

Many people would wish abortion to be easily available to ensure the safety of the woman by enabling the procedure to be carried out within a well run health system. Until well into the second half of the 20th century desperate women were sometimes forced to have abortions performed by untrained people in unhygienic conditions, and serious infections causing permanent sterility or death all too often occurred.

Morning-after pill

This pill is now available to women through family planning clinics and general practitioners. The pill is given to women who have had unprotected sexual intercourse within the past 72 hours and prevents the potentially fertilised ovum from implanting in the uterus, thus stopping the pregnancy from occurring. There has been some controversy regarding the use of the morning-after pill due to the quite acute side effects of nausea it produces, and to the ethical issues it raises for those groups who are also opposed to induced abortions.

Conclusion

Planning when to have children, and how many to have, is a matter that families take very seriously. There are many reliable methods of contraception, though it should be remembered that reliability is dependent on the contraceptives being used properly. Different methods of contraception may suit couples and families at different stages of their relationship. It is important that all couples and families have easy access to accurate and reliable information so they can choose when to have children.

It is also important to assist young people to make informed choices about sexual activity. Socio-sexual development takes place in our society many years before adolescents choose a permanent partner, or may choose to have children. The advent of HIV/AIDS and the increase in other sexually transmitted diseases such as Hepatitis B and C have implications not only for the health of the sexual partners but also for the health of their children.

Learning activities

- Find out about family planning services in your area. Is there a Family Planning Association or centre or does the local doctor or community health centre provide this service?

- Does everyone have easy access to these services? You might think about the difference between cities and rural areas.
- Collect some pamphlets on the available family planning services in your area.

Reference

Billings JJ. (1983). *The ovulation method*. Melbourne, Australian Advocate Press.

Billings EL, Westmore A. (1997). *The Billings method*. Melbourne, Anne O'Donovan.

Further reading

Clements A. Family planning. In Clements A, ed. (1992). *Infant and family health in Australia: A textbook for community health workers*. Melbourne, Churchill Livingston.

Llewellyn-Jones D. (1998). *Everywoman*. Melbourne, Penguin (9th edn.).

Publications and pamphlets from the Family Planning Association in each State and Territory.

CHAPTER 3

Having children

HAVING A CHILD is a most important event in the life of a family. The birth of a child is also the start of many years of care and responsibility through infancy, toddlerhood, the preschooler period to middle childhood, adolescence and adulthood.

Yet this care and responsibility really starts even before the pregnancy begins as the woman and her partner care for their health and are physically, emotionally and socially prepared for the pregnancy. A healthy mother provides the best possible environment for pregnancy to begin. The mother's health and lifestyle play a very important role in ensuring the health of the growing fetus.

Pregnancy

Getting pregnant

Most pregnancies are the result of sexual intercourse but there are some couples who are unable to conceive this way and for whom the technological advances of reproductive biology have been developed.

In vitro fertilisation

This literally means 'fertilisation in glass', which is where the term 'test tube baby' comes from, though in reality fertilisation takes place in a glass dish rather than a tube. *In vitro* fertilisation has been successful in helping many couples have babies.

There are some women whose fallopian tubes are blocked, thus preventing the sperm from reaching the ovum. There are many reasons why the tubes may be blocked, such as infection, ectopic pregnancies and abdominal operations.

In these cases the woman's time of ovulation is estimated and just prior to ovulation she is given a drug to help produce several ova rather than just one ovum. The ova are collected from the outer surface of the ovaries through a laparoscope and then placed in glass dishes with sperm from the male partner. The sperm are generally collected through masturbation.

The ova and sperm are closely observed for signs of fertilisation, and when this happens a decision is made as to how many fertilised ova will be put into the woman's uterus through the vagina and cervical opening. The reason why more than one fertilised ovum is usually put into the uterus is that it gives a better chance of at least one ovum implanting in the lining of the uterus and establishing a successful pregnancy. The decision as to how many fertilised ova should be put into the uterus is very complex and raises many ethical and practical issues. If too many are put in and they all implant, then the woman is likely to have a complicated pregnancy where the babies are born prematurely and may not live. On the other hand, if not enough fertilised ova are put into the uterus then none may implant and the woman and her partner have to go through the whole process again.

There are often fertilised ova that are not needed, and they are frozen. The ethical and legal aspects of who owns these ova, and when they can be used, is still being debated by ethicists, lawyers, doctors, politicians and the general community.

Artificial insemination by donor (AID)

This technique involves depositing semen from a donor male into the woman's vagina around the time of ovulation. It might be used when a male partner cannot produce any sperm (maybe because of complications from mumps as a child or for many other reasons). The couple is counselled about this procedure, as the child will not biologically be that of the mother's partner. The donated sperm usually comes from a registered sperm bank.

Lesbian couples who wish to have a child may use this procedure, though sometimes they choose to use the sperm of a trusted male friend rather than a sperm bank.

Surrogacy

This is a situation where a woman undertakes to have a baby on behalf of a couple who are unable to have a baby themselves. The surrogate mother agrees to give up all parental rights to the child in favour of that couple. The surrogate mother may be implanted with the fertilised ovum of the couple wanting the baby. This happens mainly in cases where there is something wrong with the uterus of the female partner, yet she is still producing ova. The baby is therefore biologically that of the couple and not the surrogate mother.

In other situations the surrogate mother may be artificially inseminated with sperm from the male partner of the couple wanting the baby. This generally occurs when the female partner wanting the baby is not producing ova. The baby will then be biologically that of the male partner of the couple wanting the baby, and of the surrogate mother.

Surrogacy is still fraught with problems, both legal and ethical, and there is sometimes the added emotional dilemma where the surrogate mother gives birth to the baby and finds she wishes to keep the child.

Signs and symptoms of pregnancy

The first sign of pregnancy is usually a missed period. This is a signal that the fertilised ovum has implanted in the endometrium and needs all the nutrients of the uterine lining to continue to grow. The hormonal balance in the body changes as more progesterone (a sex hormone) is needed to maintain pregnancy.

Other early signs may be swollen breasts, the need to pass urine more frequently and sometimes morning sickness.

Confirmation of pregnancy

This usually happens about 6 weeks after the last normal menstrual period. Pregnancy testing can be done with a home kit purchased from a chemist, or at a doctor's surgery or family planning clinic.

It is a very exciting time for couples, who want to share their joy with others, though some wait until the pregnancy is more established before telling many other people.

Length of pregnancy

A full-term pregnancy is 40 weeks or 9 calendar months; this is known as the gestation period. It is divided up into three stages called trimesters (which means 'three months').

The expected delivery date (EDD) or due date of a baby is calculated as a guide only and most babies do not arrive on that date but within a few days or a week either side of the EDD. Some babies arrive far too soon and they are defined as premature babies.

Fetal development

A healthy fetus needs a healthy environment within the uterus in which to develop and grow, and healthy genes from each parent to prevent harmful inherited conditions.

Normal patterns of fetal development

Up until 8 weeks after conception, the coming child is referred to as an embryo; after that it is called a fetus.

The embryo develops from the tiny cluster of cells hardly able to be seen by the naked eye at the time of conception to the baby who is born some 40 weeks later.

Here is what happens (Figure 3.1).

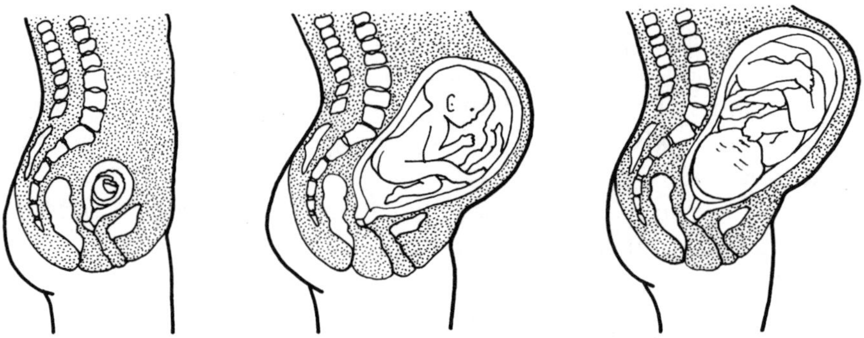

Figure 3.1 Fetal development. The embryo at 6 weeks (*left*). The fetus at 28 weeks (*centre*). The fetus at 40 weeks (*right*).

At 6 weeks

The length of the embryo is about 6 mm and the limbs are starting to bud. The diagram shows that the uterus is pushing down slightly on the mother's bladder. The mother's figure is relatively unchanged.

9 weeks

The embryo, now called a fetus, is about 3 cm and the initial structure of all internal organs is formed. The limbs are growing and there is the beginning of fingers and feet.

Eyes, ears and nostrils are well on the way.

12 weeks

The fetus is now recognisable as human. The fingers and toes can be seen and the development of ears and eyes is complete.

Most internal organs are now fully formed, including the heart. These organs now just need to grow to full size during the remainder of the pregnancy.

16 weeks

All body structures, including genitalia, are completely developed and the fetus now just needs to grow to full size. The fetus is moving within the uterus but is usually not felt by the mother until later. The fetus has started to swallow and to urinate. The length is about 18 cm and it weighs about 115 gm.

24 weeks

The mother now easily feels the fetal movements within the uterus. Some reflexes seen at birth, such as the grasp reflex, are now present. Lanugo, which is downy hair, starts to grow on the back, legs and arms. Some babies born at this stage might survive with long-term extensive special care.

28 weeks

The uterus has enlarged with the growing baby and the fundus (top of the uterus) now reaches above the mother's umbilicus (navel). The baby is moving around a lot but has not yet moved into a head-down position.

32 weeks

The baby is now usually in a head-down position. The lungs are fairly mature and the baby stands a good chance of survival if born at this stage, though special care would be needed. The baby weighs about 1.8 kg and is still very skinny, though fat under the skin now starts to form and continues to do so until birth.

40 weeks

The baby is now full-term, covered with some fat under the skin and ready to be born. The head is down in the mother's pelvis. Birthweight on average is about 3.2 kg and length is 50.8 cm.

Nutrition and removal of waste material *in utero*

The fetus gets all the nutrition and oxygen it needs, and its waste materials are removed through the mother's blood stream by way of the placenta and umbilical cord. The placenta is attached to the wall of the uterus and linked to the mother's blood circulation.

The blood carrying nutrients and oxygen goes from the mother to the placenta, where the materials needed by the baby pass into a large blood vessel in the umbilical cord and then into the circulatory system of the baby. Waste materials from the fetus go out through another blood vessel in the umbilical cord, across the placenta and into the mother's blood stream, from which it is removed through urine, sweat and breathing.

The placenta acts as a type of filter to help prevent harmful substances from getting into the fetus. However, many substances are able to cross the placenta and cause harm. This is discussed in more detail a little further on.

Amniotic sac and fluid

The developing fetus is held in the uterus in a sac (or bag) which completely encloses it. This amniotic sac (membranes) contains fluid that helps protect the fetus from any bumps that might cause injury.

The fetus is thus submerged in fluid. A white, greasy substance called vernix is formed within the uterus to protect the baby's skin in this wet environment. Babies are born still covered by vernix.

Genes and the developing fetus

The blueprint for the baby's genetic or inherited characteristics is laid down at the moment of fertilisation. Genes are inherited from both parents which may determine the child's characteristics (such as hair or eye colour or blood group) in a number of ways. Genetic conditions may be caused by single genes or groups of genes (chromosomes) which may be inherited from one or both parents, acting in combination with environmental influences.

We may have two genes (one inherited from each parent) that are the same for any given characteristic and this is known as being homozygous (homo = same zygote), or heterozygous (hetero = different zygote) when you inherit a different gene from each parent for the same characteristic. A zygote is the fertilised egg, with genes from both the male (sperm) and the female (ovum).

Genes are found on the 23 pairs of chromosomes and one of these pairs determines the sex of the fetus. Males have an X and a Y chromosome, while females have an X and an X. This means that only an X chromosome can be given by the mother, but the father can give either an X (female child) or a Y (male child) chromosome. Thus the male sperm which contains these chromosomes determines the sex of the baby.

The reader can pursue this complicated subject in more detail in Kitzinger (1997).

There are also genes for diseases. Some diseases are caused by recessive genes, where the child gets a defective gene from both parents. The parents are often heterozygous carriers, which means that the parents carry a gene for the disease without having the disease themselves. Diseases caused by recessive genes only appear when the person has two genes for that disease.

Some of these diseases are:

- Phenylketonuria (PKU), a biochemical disorder which, unless treated early, causes severe intellectual disability due to the body being unable to tolerate certain foods. Breast and cow's milk are some of these foods. The disease can be controlled by feeding the baby with soya milk and other foods that do not contain the harmful substance (phenylalanine). All babies are screened at birth by means of a simple blood test (Guthrie test), and if PKU is detected the parents are counselled and dietary information and support is given to the family.
- Cystic fibrosis, which affects the pancreas and the lungs. Children who have this disease are unable to drain the mucus away from the lungs and this causes chronic lung infections. Children whose pancreas is affected suffer from an inability to absorb food and become malnourished unless treated.
- Thalassaemia, a severe anaemia that affects people of Mediterranean and Asian origin. Treatment needs to be lifelong and regular blood transfusions may be required.

Haemophilia is a genetic disease; it is not caused by recessive genes but is sex-linked and carried on the X chromosome. The gene for the disease is carried by the female but only affects males. This disease affects the body's ability to clot blood, thus boys with this disease are at risk of bleeding badly even from a very minor injury or fall. Clotting factor can be given intravenously, which assists with the control of the disease.

The environment and fetal development

There are many environmental factors (eg. infections, toxins or nutritional problems) that can harm the fetus. Some substances are only dangerous in the first trimester while the body structures are being formed. Other substances are dangerous throughout the pregnancy.

- Rubella virus

  The rubella virus (German measles) causes damage to the developing eye, ear, brain and heart tissue if the mother contracts the disease in the first trimester of pregnancy, when these organs are being formed. Affected babies may be born with profound hearing or visual impairment, with heart defects or intellectual disabilities. Tragically, some children are affected in all these areas.

  There are now almost no children in Australia who are born with rubella-related disabilities. This is due to the immunisation programs against rubella that were initially directed at pre-teenage girls, although all children should now receive this vaccine at 12 months and before starting school.
- Smoking

  There is now clear evidence that maternal smoking harms the fetus (National Health and Medical Research Council 1997). Babies whose mothers smoked during pregnancy are much more likely to be of low birthweight and have more illnesses in infancy.
- Alcohol

  Alcohol can affect fetal development and cause Fetal Alcohol Syndrome. The baby born with this condition has some different facial features and eye folds to that of a normal baby. There may also be a mild degree of intellectual disability which is recognised as the child gets older. There is no safe level of drinking alcohol during pregnancy and pregnant women are advised to drink minimally if at all.
- Inadequate maternal diet

  A pregnant woman needs to have a diet high in protein, carbohydrates, vitamins and minerals, especially calcium. If the mother's diet is inadequate, then the nutritional needs of the fetus are not met. This may lead to a baby being born with low birthweight, even at full-term. These babies often have many problems catching up in developmental terms. Inadequate nutrition can have serious consequences for brain function and cognitive development.

  The low birthweight caused by inadequate maternal nutrition can also lead to health problems when the baby becomes an adult. Barker (1994) has suggested that full-term babies who have low birthweight may be more prone to heart disease, high blood pressure and diabetes in early adult life than those whose birthweight was normal. Work in Aboriginal communities also suggests that low birthweight may be linked to kidney disease later in life (Hoy 1997). Many Aboriginal babies are born with low birthweight, and there are very high rates of heart and kidney disease as well as diabetes among Aboriginal adults.

- Radioactivity

  In high doses such as through exposure to nuclear explosions, radiation can seriously affect fetal development and cause childhood leukaemia. Although radiation levels are low in x-rays, it is recommended that pregnant women only have x-rays if necessary for the health of the mother or baby. Female radiographers and dental nurses who work with radiation should ensure that all the occupational health and safety precautions are adhered to exactly.

- Drugs

  Many prescribed drugs may cause damage to the fetus if taken while the organs and body structures are being formed during the first trimester. Consequently, it is recommended that pregnant women do not take any drugs during this time unless there is a medical condition that must be treated with drugs known to be safe in pregnant women.

  Tragedies have occurred in the past when thalidomide (a mild sedative used to abate morning sickness) was given to pregnant women early in their pregnancy. This drug was found to affect the development of limbs and many babies were born with short limbs or no limbs at all.

  Some drugs of addiction are also dangerous to the fetus. Babies born to mothers who are heroin addicts, for example, are often born with withdrawal symptoms and may need treatment.

Interaction between genes and environment

In some instances the right environment is needed for full genetic potential to be realised. The two main examples of this interaction are:

- Height

  A baby may have the genetic potential to reach a certain height but will not do so unless the environmental conditions of full nutrition are available. A baby or young child who does not get adequate nutrition will have stunted growth.

- Intelligence

  The home, care and education environments need to be stimulating and loving. Caregivers and teachers need to provide experiences that nurture cognitive development. A child will not reach his/her full potential if he/she is unloved, neglected and given no stimulating learning experiences.

Antenatal care (care before birth)

Pregnancy and childbirth is not an illness but it is a process where complications that may harm both mother and baby can occur. It is therefore important that women and families take advantage of available antenatal care. There is clear evidence that the health of babies has improved, and maternal and child deaths have been brought to a very low rate in most of the Australian population, because pregnant women have availed themselves of antenatal care.

Aims

The main aims of antenatal care are:

- to maintain the physical, social and emotional health of the pregnant woman and her family;
- to monitor and ensure the health of the developing fetus;
- to recognise possible complications and to prevent these occurring;
- to give support to the pregnant woman and her family;
- to prepare the pregnant woman and her family for the birth of her child;
- to produce a healthy breast-fed baby;
- to prepare the family for the ongoing care of the baby after birth.

Types of antenatal care

Antenatal care is available for pregnant women and their families from:

- private specialist medical practitioners (obstetricians);
- midwives in private practice;
- general practitioners who are trained in family medicine;
- community health centres;
- public hospital outpatient departments where the care may be from a combination of medical and midwifery staff.

Other professionals involved in antenatal care are:

- physiotherapists, who help with exercises before childbirth and afterwards;
- social workers, who assist with problems the family may be experiencing;
- dietitians, who advise on adequate nutrition that is appropriate for that family;

- child-care professionals, who assist with the care of older children in the family.

The style of antenatal care chosen is not just dependent on the economic level of the family or whether they have private health insurance that would enable them to go to a private obstetrician. Many families feel much more at ease with a midwife, whom they get to know over the months and who can give the families the time that is needed to discuss questions and concerns. Experienced midwives will always refer the mother and family to a specialist if potential complications arise.

Health care

If the pregnancy has been confirmed by a home test kit, the pregnant woman should see a medical practitioner or midwife soon afterwards.

At this visit her personal and family history will be noted so that any obvious risks to the baby or mother can be assessed. This assessment should also look at the social, emotional and cultural needs of the woman and her family.

Other tests at this initial visit will include blood screening to identify her blood group and also whether it is rhesus positive or negative. Rubella immunity is also checked.

Ongoing visits to health-care professionals

Patterns of health visits after the initial visit may differ for individual women but will usually include:

- every 4 weeks until 28–30 weeks
- every 2 weeks from 30–36 weeks
- every week from 36 weeks to delivery.

Health-care checks

There are various aspects of the pregnancy that need to be checked each visit. These are:

- general health of the mother and family;
- weight of the mother—too much weight can be a sign of complications;
- height of the fundus (top) of the uterus—this is a guide to the size of the fetus;
- blood pressure of the mother—a rise in blood pressure may signal complications;
- urine test—protein in the urine is a sign of complications;

- any swelling of the ankles or other parts of the body, especially in late pregnancy;
- fetal heart beat after about 14–16 weeks, using a special stethoscope;
- haemoglobin level of mother to check that she is getting enough iron.

Other tests done may include an ultrasound, which gives clear evidence of the baby's growth, size and position. Some problems of pregnancy, such as when the placenta is placed too low in the uterus, will be recognised on an ultrasound. This means that measures can be taken to prevent further complications and to ensure the safest birth plan is decided upon.

Some women may also have a glucose tolerance test during pregnancy to see if they are able to clear glucose (sugar) from their body. This is to find out if the woman has gestational diabetes, which we will discuss a little further on.

Pregnancy and birth care plan

One of the criticisms of antenatal care has been that it was too clinical and had not involved the woman and family enough in decision making. Doctors might do some tests, give some instructions, and the women would go away feeling as though her body and her baby did not belong to her.

Women are now encouraged to involve their partners and families in deciding what is best for them during their pregnancy and through childbirth, too. Family background, personal values and cultural factors all play an important part in this decision making.

Diet

This is of crucial importance to the health of the mother and the baby. The woman needs to ensure that she has a well balanced diet with adequate amounts of protein and calcium for the tissues and bones of the growing fetus. Foods high in iron are also needed, as the woman's own supply can become depleted due to the demands of the fetus. Extra iron and calcium in the form of tablets are sometimes prescribed.

Foods high in vitamin B are very important and studies have shown that there is less risk of neural tubal defects (spina bifida) if the mother's diet contains high amounts of folates, a type of vitamin B (Bower 1993). All green leafy vegetables are high in folates. Folate supplements in tablet form may be recommended one month before and 3 months after conception for all women, but especially those where there is a family history of neural tube defects.

Exercise

Keeping fit is very important during pregnancy and exercises such as walking and swimming are very suitable. Many women find it easy to maintain their pre-pregnancy exercise pattern. Athletes and sportswomen who train heavily may need to restrict their level of activity and should seek medical advice regarding this.

Emotional and social care

Antenatal care should include the whole family and the preparation of other children for the birth of a sibling. Older children can share what is happening during the pregnancy while younger children, especially toddlers, need special understanding during this time and when the baby is born.

Families also need support in the changes that happen, with first babies in particular. These changes may be financial as the couple go from two incomes to only one. The changes may be social, as many mothers choose to go on maternity leave which means a change in lifestyle from working outside the home to the full-time care of a small baby. Some families may decide that the father will be the main caregiver and this will need social and emotional adjustments for the couple.

Preparation for birth

This is a most important part of antenatal care, which both partners can share. Childbirth has been, for many women, a rather frightening experience because they were really unsure of what was happening. Labour wards tended to be overbright and noisy, with the partner banished, and a lack of explanation given to the woman. She often felt alone, abandoned and scared.

Childbirth education programs, which are held by hospitals and some non-government organisations, have been responsible for improving the experience for families during the birth of their baby. These groups have also helped health professionals become more attuned to what families want and need during pregnancy and childbirth.

The programs give detailed explanations of what happens during labour and birth. There are also exercise programs to assist with breathing and relaxation during and between contractions. Partners or support persons share these exercise programs, so that there is a shared anticipation and appreciation of what will happen. Visits are also arranged to the hospital so that the setting, equipment and staff are familiar, or at least less strange. Preparation for breastfeeding is also discussed, and what to expect after the baby's birth.

These groups often have a social benefit, too, as couples meet each other and share experiences. This sharing may extend to well after the birth and be the start of lasting friendship and support as the families grow.

Cultural factors play a large part in a partner's willingness and ability to be involved in childbirth education or the birth itself. In some cultures having a baby is seen very much to be women's business and it would be intrusive and inappropriate for a male to become involved. It is usually permissible for a sister, mother, or mother-in-law to be the support person.

Some complications of pregnancy

Ectopic or tubal pregnancy

This occurs when the fertilised ovum implants itself in the fallopian tube instead of the uterus. The woman has all the usual signs and symptoms of pregnancy and her periods stop due to the hormonal changes.

An ectopic pregnancy is a potentially serious condition as the growing embryo can become too big for the fallopian tube, causing the tube to burst and bleed into the abdominal cavity. This is an emergency situation and without immediate surgery the woman could die. She may become infertile, as the fallopian tubes may be damaged.

Gestational diabetes

Some women develop diabetes during pregnancy, which means that they are unable to clear sugar from their bodies. A possible complication of this is that the baby can become very large, which is not healthy and makes a normal vaginal delivery very difficult. Gestational diabetes also increases the risk of the fetus developing other abnormalities.

Women who develop gestational diabetes are put on a strict, but healthy, diet with controlled quantities of carbohydrates spread regularly through the day.

Pre-eclampsia

This condition is a warning that all is not going well and that the mother is not getting rid of all the baby's waste materials from her body. Consequently the mother gets swollen ankles, high blood pressure and protein in her urine, which are signs her kidneys are not coping.

The aim of the treatment is to prevent the pre-eclampsia from progressing to eclampsia (toxaemia) which is very serious and can cause the death of both the mother and the baby. Drugs to lower blood pressure are often prescribed. Strict bed rest and even hospitalisation may be necessary in some cases. The signs and symptoms are monitored carefully, and if they persist or get worse labour will be induced early in order to prevent damage being done to mother or baby. Pre-eclampsia usually occurs in the latter stages of pregnancy, so the baby has a very good chance of survival.

Birth

Nearly all babies born in Australia today are born in a hospital setting, though an increasing number of couples are choosing to have their baby at home. Couples should be aware of the options, and the benefits and dangers of each place of birth, so that they can make a decision based on accurate information.

Hospital birth

Labour room

These are rooms within the maternity section of a public or private hospital that are set up for the birth of a baby, with all the necessary equipment and staff to cope if an emergency or complication should arise. Women are moved from the maternity ward to the labour room just before the birth of the baby. Labour rooms are very clinical, though the style of furnishings and attitudes of the staff have made them much more friendly than they were in the past.

Birthing centre

These are rooms furnished in a relaxed style where there is room for partners and other family members or friends to stay and where the couple can feel more at home than in a maternity ward or labour room setting. Birth takes place in this relaxed setting. These centres are usually run by midwives.

Birthing centres are usually attached to a maternity hospital so that complications, if they arise, can be treated by an obstetrician and emergency care is available if it becomes necessary. Women who give birth in these centres are assessed during pregnancy to be at low risk of any complications.

Home birth

Having their baby at home in familiar and loved surroundings is very appealing to many couples and some doctors and midwives are supportive of this wish. It is easy to understand the emotional reasons for wanting a home birth.

The emotional need of the couple should be balanced with the need to safeguard the health and safety of both the mother and child. Women who plan to have their baby at home will have a very careful assessment as to the potential possibilities of any complications, and back-up support would be arranged in case of unforeseen emergencies.

Many babies are born safely at home, as shown by a Western Australian study (Woodcock 1994), which compared hospital and home births. It is logical to expect fewer complications in home births when all the women with potential complications are referred to a hospital setting. However, it should be remembered that some babies whose mothers have been assessed as low-risk have died during home birth in Australia over the past ten years, even when attended by experienced midwives or doctors.

The three stages of birth

First stage

This stage is from the start of the first uterine contraction to the time when the cervix of the uterus is fully dilated. It can be quite a long drawn-out stage, as the contractions may start very slowly and the baby's head may take some time to get into position for birth. The cervix may also dilate very slowly. The first stage of labour is usually much longer with first babies than with subsequent births and may last for more than 12 hours. There is a careful monitoring of both mother and baby so that if signs of fetal distress are noted, appropriate steps can immediately be taken.

Women usually need much psychological and physical support during this stage, as it can be very tiring. This support is best given by the partner or other chosen person. A woman who has a birth plan and who has been to childbirth preparation classes will nearly alway find this of enormous help, as she and her partner know what to expect and have learnt useful ways of breathing and relaxing during and between contractions. Many women find it helpful to have hot showers or baths during this time, as the heat soothes the pain.

The pain of contractions is often very severe, so many women use gas (nitrous oxide) as relief. Others may choose stronger analgesia such as pethidine. Other women will decide on an epidural injection, where an anaesthetic is put into the space around the spinal cord in the lower back. This anaesthetic stops all the pain of contractions, while the woman is still alert for the birth of the baby.

The membranes often break (usually referred to as 'the waters breaking') at the end of the first stage, although it can happen much earlier and may even be the first sign that labour is beginning.

Second stage

This stage is the birth of the baby. The woman generally needs to assist here by pushing to get the head and one shoulder out, and the rest of the baby generally comes easily after that. This, of course, is the time that everyone has been waiting for and is a very close moment for the parents of the new baby or for the mother and her support person. This closeness can be there even when there are hospital staff attending to the mother and baby.

The baby is placed on the mother's chest and both parents can stroke their new son or daughter. Babies do not always cry immediately at birth and there is no concern if the baby is breathing well and his or her colour is good. Medical or nursing staff will immediately check the baby's physical condition by taking an Apgar score, which is a series of quick observations that note colour, responses, breathing, muscle tone and heart beat. This is done immediately after birth and again 5 minutes later. Babies with a low Apgar score need to be observed very carefully and may need resuscitation and special care.

The umbilical cord is still attached to the baby and it is best to wait until it has stopped beating before it is clamped and cut. This helps the baby get all the nutrients possible from the mother. The father or support person may be the one to cut the cord. There are no nerve endings in the umbilical cord, so cutting it does not hurt the baby. A baby may be given an injection of vitamin K to assist with the blood clotting.

Third stage

The placenta is expelled at this stage, which usually happens a few minutes after the baby is born. An injection of ergometrine, which helps contract the walls of the blood vessels, is often given to the mother just prior to this stage. Occasionally there are complications where the cord breaks or the placenta does not separate from the wall of the uterus and may need to be surgically removed. The placenta is examined, as it gives evidence of the health of the baby within the uterus.

Episiotomy

Sometimes a doctor or midwife will cut the back part of the vagina at the start of second stage in order to help the baby's head get out. This is called an episiotomy and will be sewn up once the placenta has been expelled. This is thought to be less traumatic to the mother than a tear in the vaginal wall caused by pressure from the baby's head.

Complications of birth

Position of baby

The normal position of babies prior to birth is that of head-down, with the curve of the back in the curve of the mother's abdomen and forming the main part of the bulge.

Babies do sometimes get themselves into very different, and difficult, positions with their bottoms and legs being down low and heads up high, which is called a breech position. Other babies lie sideways across the uterus and have no way of being born at all. Babies in difficult positions need help to be born and that can be by caesarean section or with the help of forceps.

Caesarean section

There are many reasons other than difficult positions why babies are unable to be born by normal vaginal delivery. It may be that the placenta is placed too low down and the mother might haemorrhage if birth occurred through the vagina. The mother may be in labour and her cervix not dilating when fetal distress is observed.

In both these cases a Caesarean section would be performed, where the baby is born through an incision through the mother's abdominal wall.

Having a Caesarean section does not mean that the parents cannot share the birth. Modern anaesthesia allows women to have the operation under a local epidural anaesthetic so she is wide awake and can see the baby immediately after it is taken from her uterus. Partners sometimes share this experience and, even if not in the room, the partner is given the baby soon after birth.

Forceps delivery

Forceps are sometimes used when the baby's head needs a little bit of help during second stage. They may be used to assist a baby in breech position where the bottom is coming out first, or where the baby is very small.

Induction of labour

There are some situations where it would be unwise for the pregnancy to continue any further. It may be that the mother is ill or at risk of toxaemia, or that the baby has stopped growing or that the placenta is no longer transferring nutrients.

In these cases the labour is induced artificially by rupturing the membranes and then giving hormones that cause the uterus to contract. The hormones are usually given by intravenous infusion (drip).

Immediately after the birth: The neonatal period

After the baby is born

The newborn baby is, as mentioned before, placed immediately on the mother's abdomen or chest, usually with skin-to-skin contact. The medical or nursing staff will have taken an Apgar score, and if all is well the baby will spend some time with the parents before other examinations are done.

This is an important time. It is the first time the baby is a completely separate person, the first time the parents have seen the baby, the first time the baby and parents have had external contact such as stroking. This is a getting-to-know-each-other time, a time of bonding, and should not be hurried. Some mothers find their feelings confused at this time and should be reassured that it is very natural to need to get to know the new baby.

The baby will be still wet from the amniotic fluid and may have some bloodstains from the mother's vagina. There will still be some vernix covering the baby and perhaps the head will seem a little out of shape, which is quite normal. The baby may still have a covering of downy hair over her body. (To avoid using terms like 'him/her', 'he/she' etc. we shall assume from this point on that our baby is a girl.)

The room should be warm enough, as the newborn baby now has to control her own body temperature and will lose heat quickly if the room is too cool.

The baby will usually be bathed after she and the parents (or mother and support person) have spent some time getting to know each other. It is usually the father who baths the baby for this first time, and babies usually relax in the water as though they have returned to the familiar watery damp of the uterus.

Measurements

Now is the time for the weighing and measuring. The main measurements taken are:

- Weight or body mass, which in most healthy full-term babies will be approximately 3–3.5 kg. There are considerable individual differences: large parents tend to have larger babies, smaller parents may have smaller babies, and girls are often smaller than boys.
- Length, which averages about 50 cm.
- Head circumference, which should be about 35 cm.

These measurements are important, not just at birth but because they also provide a reference point for growth patterns in infancy.

The newborn baby

The newborn baby (neonate) is now in a very different environment. Some of these differences include:

- the change from being immersed in amniotic fluid to the entry into air;
- the change from receiving oxygen from the mother to breathing independently;
- the change from obtaining nourishment through the mother to taking external nourishment;
- the change from excreting waste products through the mother to independently eliminating waste products from the body;
- the need to maintain body temperature independently from the mother.

Reflexes

The baby does not come into the world totally unprepared. The normal body functions such as breathing and excreting start working at birth and the baby has many protective and other reflexes that are automatic. These reflexes are also a sign that the baby's nervous system is well developed and working properly. Most reflexes are apparent for a limited time and their disappearance is also an indication that the nervous system is developing as it should.

Sucking reflex

All healthy babies are born with the ability to suck and will suck anything that is put in their mouth. Most babies start sucking on the mother's breast immediately after birth. This sucking is important as it assists with bonding between mother and child and it also gives the baby colostrum, the fluid secreted before breast milk. The sucking reflex lasts until the baby is about 4 months old when awake, and 7 months when asleep.

Seeking reflex (sometimes called rooting reflex)

This reflex allows a baby to find the mother's nipple to suck. The stroking of the baby's cheek will find the baby automatically turning to that side to seek the nipple. Mothers who try to turn the baby's head toward the breast by pushing the outside cheek will find the baby turns the opposite way. The seeking reflex lasts until the baby is 3 to 4 months of age.

Moro reflex

Any sudden movement of the neck backwards will cause the baby to jerk her arms outwards and then to move them together. This is a protective mechanism, showing that the baby is aware of the danger of falling. The reflex disappears by 3 to 4 months of age.

Startle reflex

This is very similar to the Moro reflex, but happens with sudden loud noises.

Grasp reflex

A newborn baby will firmly grasp objects that touch her palm. This reflex has gone by 3 to 4 months of age.

Plantar reflex

This is rather like a grasp reflex of the toes, where the toes curl under if the sole of the foot is touched. The baby shows this reflex until 8 to 12 months of age.

Walking reflex

A newborn baby will, if held upright with her legs on a firm surface, move her legs in a walking motion. The reflex lasts until 2 to 3 months of age.

Senses of the neonate

Newborn babies also use many of their senses in starting to understand about the world into which they have been born.

Sight

Babies can see at birth, though only for short distances. There is some evidence that they prefer human faces to other sights. This is a very sensible preference, as the baby needs humans to provide care, security and nourishment. Newborn babies also react to light, and will close their eyes if the light is very bright.

Hearing

A baby will blink eyes or open them widely if there is a sudden sound. After a few days they seem to respond to their mother's voice and may quieten for a short time when she talks.

Smell

Babies recognise the smell of milk and can probably recognise their mother's smell by about 10 days of age.

Taste

Babies definitely prefer sweet tastes to sour or bitter ones. Breast milk is high in lactose, which is milk sugar, so they get used to a sweet taste very quickly.

Touch

Newborn babies certainly respond to pain and discomfort and will be comforted when cuddled and rocked. They will soon start to explore their world by mouthing and by feeling objects.

Feeding in the neonatal period

The establishment of breastfeeding is a major aim over the first few days after birth. Breastfeeding is a very natural act yet it does need to be learnt, so it is best for the mother to have prepared prior to birth and to have skilled and supportive care after the birth.

The baby has her first fumbling sucks immediately after birth. This helps bond mother and child and it also gives the baby some colostrum, a substance secreted before the milk comes in. Colostrum is important because it contains vitamins for nutrition and antibodies for fighting infection. The newborn baby has very few defences against infection and needs all the help she can get.

Sucking soon after birth encourages commencement of lactation. The hormonal balance of the mother's body during and after birth trigger lactation, but the more the baby sucks, the more milk the mother will secrete.

The baby is born with lots of fluid in her tissues and is also rather tired due to the effort of getting out into the world, so she sleeps a lot over the first couple of days. When awake she should be put to the breast even though the mother's milk supply is not yet established.

Breastfeeding is a time for physical closeness and for bonding. It should be taken gently so that the mother does not get anxious about feeding the baby. Attaching the baby to the breast needs care. The baby needs to put her mouth right around the nipple and coloured area (areola) of the breast rather than sucking just the nipple. Babies need practice at this and a slow, gentle start is best.

Many babies snort a lot at the start of feeding because they cannot breathe through their mouth while sucking, so need a clear airway for their nose which sometimes gets pushed against the fullness of the mother's breast and blocks off the airway. Unable to breathe, the baby keeps releasing the breast from the mouth and then has to attach all over again. This problem can generally be prevented by ensuring the baby has a clear airway to the nose, which the mother does by pressing her breast at the point where it is near the baby's nose.

All women are encouraged to breast feed and should be given enough information and support to allow this to happen. Many professional organisations such as the Public Health Association of Australia and the Australian Early Childhood Association have formal policies aimed at promoting and maintaining breastfeeding. Community organisations such as the Nursing Mothers' Association of Australia are able to give ongoing support and information to breastfeeding mothers.

A special note

Breastfeeding is actively encouraged, but some women find breastfeeding difficult and/or distasteful. The woman's feelings must be respected and there should be no feelings of guilt induced or disapproval shown. Every assistance must be given to establish bottle feeding with a formula that suits the baby. Clear instructions must be given to the mother about the importance of sterility and correct strength of formula so that she is confident about feeding her baby.

Advantages of breastfeeding

- Breast milk contains all the nutrients a baby needs, in the correct strength and of the correct type. The sugars, protein and fats, mineral salts and vitamins are all nutritionally ideal for the baby.
- Breast milk contains antibodies from the mother which help fight infection. The newborn and young baby has very little resistance to infection, so that getting some of the mother's protection against disease through the breast milk is important.
- Breast milk needs no preparation or sterilisation. This means that the risk of infection is much reduced.
- Breast milk comes at the right temperature for the baby.
- Breastfeeding helps the uterus return to its non-pregnant size.
- Breastfeeding encourages closeness between mother and baby, and this is important for bonding.

- Breastfeeding is convenient and available at any time. There is no need to prepare bottles and worry about having enough when mother and baby are away from home.

Are there any disadvantages with breastfeeding?

There are no real disadvantages with breastfeeding if the mother is healthy, though there are two points worth noting:

- Some mothers still feel uneasy about breastfeeding in public, but community awareness of the importance of breastfeeding is helping to make this less of an issue.
- Breastfeeding can only be given by the mother and not shared by the father or other family members, although even this is changing. The advent of efficient breast pumps and the availability of domestic deep-freezing facilities have meant that the mother can easily express milk to be frozen and given in a bottle at a later stage. There are freeze packs designed especially for expressed breast milk, which makes this process relatively simple. Parents may bring such packs to child care for the staff to give to the baby during the day. This will be discussed in more detail in Chapter 8.

Contraindications to breastfeeding

There are some situations where it is unwise to breast feed. These are:

- When the mother is ill and being treated with drugs that might be secreted in the breast milk and harm the baby.
- If the mother is HIV positive, the virus can be transmitted to the baby. In Australia mothers would be advised to bottle feed using a suitable formula, and assistance would be given to ensure this was successful. In Africa this is a real dilemma. The breastfed baby of an HIV-positive mother may also become HIV-positive. The bottle-fed baby in poor areas of Africa has a high chance of dying from malnutrition or diarrhoeal disease within the first few months.

Possible early problems with breastfeeding

Babies suck very hard and some mothers get cracked and sore nipples in the early stages of breastfeeding. This can be very painful. Some preventive measures include:

- preparation of nipples in pregnancy, though studies indicate that this does not help;

- ensuring that the baby's mouth is in the correct position while feeding;
- the use of nipple shields until the nipples become tougher.

Some mothers get engorged breasts, which are not only very painful but can also become infected (mastitis) and need antibiotic treatment. Various creams have been tried to relieve the pain of engorgement. Another suggested treatment is the use of cold cabbage leaves on the breasts (Roberts 1995). Ice packs may also help relieve the pain.

Wind

Babies tend to suck air into their stomach while feeding, though this happens a lot less with breast-fed babies. The air causes wind in the baby's digestive system and this leads to abdominal pain. It is standard practice with babies to sit them upright and gently rub their back until they burp. Some parents prefer to hold the baby over a shoulder and pat the baby's back. It is wise to have a protective cloth in place, as the baby is very likely to burp up some milk onto the shoulder on which she is lying.

Posetting

It is very common for babies to regurgitate some milk after they have been fed. Parents should not worry about this if the amount is small. Advice should be sought if the amount is large or if the vomiting is projectile, as this is a sign of pyloric stenosis where the muscle at the bottom of the stomach will not open and allow food to get through to the small intestine.

Frequency of feeding

Generally, babies are the best judge of when they are hungry and need feeding. Mothers soon get used to the cries that signal that a baby is hungry rather than tired or uncomfortable. A healthy baby should be fed when she signals she is hungry and fed for as long as it takes for her to feel full. She will then stop sucking and usually fall asleep looking very relaxed and contented.

The only situation where babies need special feeding times is if the baby is unwell and is too sleepy to feed without being roused. These babies should be under supervision of a nurse or medical practitioner who can assist the mother with feeding routines.

Care of the newborn

The neonatal period is very much a transitional time: a time between womb and the world as it were. It is a time when the baby establishes feeding and other body functions, when bonds with other family members—which have begun before birth—are strengthened. Mother and baby get to know each other, with support from family and health-care staff. All babies are different, and each has an individual personality with different likes and dislikes, which mothers often recognise from the time of the baby's birth (Sheridan 1993).

The neonatal period is also used to assess physical health and give any assistance with practical care that might be needed.

Weight

The baby's weight is monitored to ensure that all is going well. Babies lose excess fluid from their bodies over the first few days, which means they lose weight after birth. They quickly regain this once they have begun feeding.

Physical examination

A careful examination of the baby will be carried out, usually by a paediatrician (a specialist in child health) or trainee paediatrician.

- The general appearance of the baby is observed, the colour and feel of the skin, the way the baby is lying, the state of alertness.
- The reflexes will be checked to assess the competency of the nervous system.
- Eyes and ears are examined.
- Sight and hearing are checked.
- Abdominal organs are gently palpated to check for any abnormality.
- The hips are rotated to check for any signs of dislocation, which some babies do have at birth. Unnoticed and untreated, the condition can hinder walking.
- Hands and feet are checked for signs of Down syndrome or club foot.
- The spine is checked for any signs of spina bifida.
- Genitalia and anus are checked for any abnormality.
- The heart sounds and breathing are examined.
- The mouth is examined for any signs that the palate has not properly developed.

- Elimination processes of passing urine and bowel motions are checked. The first bowel motion passed by the baby is greeny-black in colour and called meconium.
- Feeding is checked.

Screening

All babies in Australia have a Guthrie test from a heel prick of blood to check for hidden diseases such as phenylketonuria (PKU), the genetic metabolic disease discussed earlier. Babies who are positive for this test will need to be fed soya milk initially and go onto a special diet when weaned or introduced to solids. Parents of these babies will need counselling regarding the condition and the chances of further children being affected. Other diseases checked for at this stage are:

- congenital hypothyroidism, which is a cause of intellectual disability;
- cystic fibrosis (see Chapter 10);
- galactosaemia, where certain substances in milk are not metabolised.

Immunisation

From May 2000, all babies born in Australia are given the first dose of hepatitis B vaccine before leaving hospital. This is necessary because of the rising rate of hepatitis B in the community.

Babies in all States and Territories are immunised for specific diseases after birth if their mother has a disease such as tuberculosis or hepatitis B.

Cord care

The umbilical cord stump needs to be observed to ensure that it is drying out well and that there is no sign of infection or bleeding. It may be gently cleaned with an antiseptic lotion each day after bathtime. The stump usually falls off several days after birth.

Some characteristics of the newborn

Fontanelles

A baby's skull needs to grow very fast in the first year so that the brain can grow. The baby is therefore born with a strong membrane rather than bone over part of the brain at the top and back of the head. The fontanelle at the top of the head actually grows for the first 2 to 3 months after birth and then usually slowly closes between 12 and 18 months. The fontanelle at the back of the head, which is much smaller than that at the front, usually closes after 2 months. Care needs to be taken of the baby's head during routines such as bathing.

Jaundice

Some babies develop jaundice, where the skin becomes a yellow colour, soon after birth. This is because the liver, which gets rid of many toxins in the body, has not yet started to function properly. In most cases where the baby is full-term the jaundice is fairly mild and may be treated by placing the baby under ultra-violet light for a period each day. The eyes of the baby are protected during this treatment.

Skin pigmentation

Babies are often born with patches of skin that are pink or darker than the usual skin colour. These are referred to as birthmarks and often fade within a few months. Others persist for some years or even throughout life. Many babies have pink marks over their eyelids that are called 'stork marks'; these generally fade within a few months.

There may be a largish patch of greyish-blue pigmentation over the area of the lower back. This colouring is called a Mongolian blue spot and is found in nearly all non-white babies and in some white babies. It usually disappears after 2 or 3 years. Care needs to be taken that these spots are not confused with bruising.

Breasts and genitalia

The genitals of both males and females are larger at birth compared with the rest of the body. This is perfectly normal. Maternal hormones cross the placenta into the baby at birth, so genitals may get larger after birth and breast enlargement may occur. This enlargement and swelling resolves itself in the days after birth.

Circumcision of male babies

This procedure, which involves cutting the foreskin off the tip of the penis, was once almost routine for male babies and was usually done a few days after birth. There is a risk of subsequent severe bleeding and infection that can cause serious illness and occasionally death. There is no obvious health benefit from the procedure, though there are current discussions going on as to whether non-circumcised males are more at risk of contracting sexually transmitted diseases and urinary tract infections. Circumcision in some health settings is actively discouraged except where it has cultural or religious significance, as for example in Jewish families.

There are some parents who would wish it to be done for family and personal reasons and this wish should be respected and discussed and the dangers to the baby pointed out. There are many doctors who will not perform circumcision unless there is a medical reason for doing so.

If circumcision is performed, then care of the penis is similar to that of the cord site: keeping the wound clean and dry and preventing bleeding and infection.

Parents and the baby

Post-natal period

The post-natal (after birth) period, which is from birth to 6 weeks of age, is very important for the health of both the baby and family. The mother and other family members need to feel confident about the practical care of the baby before they leave hospital. In the case of early discharge from hospital, or a home birth, there should be domiciliary health staff who visit the mother at home to provide support and advice.

Bathing and dressing

Some parents feel quite anxious about bathing their baby for the first time and worry about the baby being slippery and hard to hold. These fears should be taken seriously and assistance given so that confidence is gained. Practical advice as to how to wash the hair and face first and the use of non-slippery solutions in the bath water rather than soap is a way of helping confidence develop.

Bathtime is a lovely time for parents and the baby. Most babies really enjoy the freedom and relaxation of kicking in the warm water. So it is a time for enjoyment, not just for getting clean.

Babies do not like having their faces covered and will cry loudly if this happens, so it is important to dress the baby without causing distress. The design of clothes with wide neck openings, as well as giving parents tips such as getting the face through first, are both ways of keeping the baby comfortable.

Discussion with parents about safety during bathtime, dressing and nappy changing is very important. Babies should never be left alone in a bath or on a changing table for even a moment.

Nappy changing

Most parents quickly become competent at this routine and may work out ways to share dealing with the dirty nappies. The importance of changing frequently in order to prevent nappy rash is pointed out, as is the need to carefully wipe away all urine and faeces from the skin. The wiping motion should be from front to back in the case of girls so that the vaginal and urethral area is not contaminated with faeces.

The choice of nappies to be used is a decision that is influenced by lifestyle and personal preference. Disposable nappies are certainly convenient, though they are expensive and there is no totally satisfactory method of disposal. Most people wrap them up and put them in the rubbish tin, which can be unpleasant in a warm climate.

Cloth nappies require an initial expenditure on purchase and ongoing cleaning, soaking, washing and drying. Some parents decide on a combination of nappies: cloth nappies at home and disposables when out or travelling.

Many people have objected to disposable nappies on environmental grounds. It may well be, though, that more energy is used, and pollution caused, by the chemicals used to soak and wash cloth nappies and the electricity needed to heat water to wash and dry them than is used to make the disposable variety. There are, however, still no satisfactory solutions to the break-down of the plastic content of disposable nappies.

Baby massage

This has been part of infant care in many cultures for a long, long time and is now accepted practice in Australia. The gentle rubbing of a suitable oil onto the baby's body not only relaxes the baby but also provides tactile (touch) and olfactory (smell) stimulation and enhances the physical contact between mother (or other family member) and child.

Feeding and sleeping patterns

Newborn babies tend to sleep, and wake only to feed. The periods of wakefulness get longer as babies get older. The mother and baby may take some time to get their sleep patterns together. Feeling tired is one of the concerns of nearly all mothers of young babies.

General reassurance

The social and emotional health of the family are very important, as the baby's care depends on the family's wellbeing. Having time to get to know the new baby, to hold and to touch, is an important part of initial infant care. Parents need reassurance about many aspects of care, and questions about small matters or concerns should be responded to with sensitivity and respect.

Some parental concerns

'Baby blues'

Many women feel rather miserable and often weepy about the third day after birth. This is due to the changing hormones in their bodies, but it is often hard for the woman and her partner to understand what is happening. Here they are, the proud parents of a new baby, and the mother keeps bursting into tears! Explanation and understanding should be given to both parents. In most cases, the situation quickly resolves itself but there is always the danger that a more serious and long-lasting post-natal depression can occur.

Post-natal depression

This is a potentially serious condition that may affect the mother's ability to care for the baby, and nearly always disrupts the developing relationship between mother and child. In severe cases, post-natal depression may lead the mother to harm the child. The cause is unknown, though some women appear to be at more risk of developing post-natal depression than others.

Many women do not seek help for their depression because they do not recognise their feelings. It is also hard for many women to admit they have difficulty in coping with a new baby. Child-care staff can help by sensitive listening and being aware of both verbal and non-verbal cues that might indicate that all is not well with the mother.

Colic

Some babies have a period of restless, red-faced crying where they pull their legs up in a position that shows they are in pain. This is called colic and often happens at the end of the day or early evening. This is usually the busiest time of the day, when the evening meal is being prepared and other children need attention.

Many, many experts have given explanations as to why this happens but no one has come up with a preventive measure or with a way of stopping the pain or the crying. Holding, rocking and walking the baby may only give relief for a few moments or minutes. The crying may last up to 2 or more hours and is very distressing for the whole family.

Families can be given the reassurance that colic generally disappears by 3 months, though this is scarcely a comfort at evening meal time, when a toddler is demanding food, an older child needs attention and the baby is screaming. Many families work out a way of both partners being available during the colic period of the day so that the stress can be shared.

Safety issues

Parents frequently request advice about ways of keeping baby safe. The decision about the type of clothing, bedding and nursery furniture is usually made before birth, as is the type of restraint to be fitted into the car. Most parents these days use baby capsules that clamp into a fitting in the car and can be easily taken out and used as a carry basket. Advice about safe nursery equipment and toys can be obtained from Kidsafe (Child Accident Prevention Foundation of Australia), who have divisions in each State and Territory. Child safety will be discussed in detail in Chapter 8.

Sudden infant death syndrome (SIDS or cot death)

The unexpected death of a healthy baby is, of course, totally devastating and tragic for the parents and family. Much research has been carried out but no one definite cause has been found. A number of risk factors have, however, been identified. These are:

- smoking during pregnancy;
- smoking in the home of the baby;
- babies lying on their tummy;
- babies being too hot or too cold;
- over-dressing or over-covering the baby with blankets.

It is therefore recommended that:

- babies are put to sleep on their side or back;
- no-one smokes in the home, and that babies are not taken to smoky places;
- babies are not overdressed or have too many bed covers;
- the baby's head stays uncovered during sleep;
- rooms are not overheated or too cold. (Henderson-Smart et al. 1998).

These recommendations apply to child-care settings as much as to homes. The rate of SIDS in Australia has been reduced since these recommendations were promoted.

Going home with the new baby

The family will have ongoing assistance from professionals to ensure the continuing health of the family and baby. Often this takes the form of a visit to the home by a community-health nurse and then the family visits the child and family health centre. Each State and Territory has these facilities, though they may be called by different names.

The health of the mother is monitored as well as that of the baby. The baby is regularly weighed and feeding patterns are discussed. Immunisation and other health promotion information is given to parents. There is also the opportunity to talk about any problems or concerns.

Many child and family-health centres hold coffee mornings where the parents (mainly mothers) get to know each other and share child-rearing experiences.

Sibling adjustment

The ease with which other children in the family settle down with the new baby is often to do with age. Children over the age of 4, or those who already have a sibling, are usually excited and happy to welcome the new baby.

A 2-year-old who has had his parents to himself, and who is still finding sharing a difficult concept, may show some anxiety about the new baby and may even want to pinch or bite the new sibling who seems to have taken over from him. This is very understandable behaviour, as is that of the toddler who shows signs of developmental regression by wanting a bottle again or wetting his pants when he was previously going to the toilet.

The toddler here needs lots of attention; he needs to know his parents still love him and gradually there will be acceptance of the baby. Child-care staff can often assist parents by being understanding of the toddler's needs at this time. Reassurance for the parents that the toddler's behaviour is very usual is helpful too.

Blended families

Tact and sensitivity needs to be shown where one of the parents has children from another marriage or relationship. Children from the former relationship sometimes feel disloyal to the parent who is no longer part of that relationship. This can happen when parents separate and divorce and the children live with their mother. The father forms another relationship and has a child. The older children may be delighted with their new half-sibling but be concerned that their attitude may show disloyalty to their mother.

Other situations

Premature babies

Some babies are born well before their due date and need special care. There are many reasons for babies being born prematurely, which include ill health or injury to the mother, though there are often no obvious reasons.

The intensity of the special care needed generally depends on the prematurity of the baby. A baby born at 36 weeks who weighs just over 2 kg will not need as much special care as the baby of 27 weeks who does not even weigh 1 kg.

The internal organs of premature babies, especially the lungs, have not grown enough for independent function. The sucking reflex is not strong, so the baby needs feeding through a tube and needs to be given assistance to breathe. The environment of the premature baby needs to one where the temperature is constant and the humidity increased, so these babies are placed in special humidicribs within a special-care neonatal nursery that has the technology and trained staff to ensure the best care of the baby.

Yet technology and trained staff alone are not enough. These babies need physical contact with their parents, even if they are too small and sick to be taken out of the humidicrib. Mothers are encouraged to sit with their baby and to stroke and touch often. The humidicribs have special side openings to allow this to happen. Talking quietly and soft singing is also encouraged.

Breast milk is important for these babies. The mother expresses milk as soon as she can and the baby is then given this milk. Expressing milk also helps establish lactation so the baby can start to breast feed when she is strong enough.

Multiple births

Two percent of deliveries are of twins. Triplets and other multiple births occur much more rarely. Multiple births do run in the family, so the chance of having more than one baby is higher if there are twins on either side of the family. IVF is also likely to give multiple births. There are two types of naturally occurring twins.

Monozygotic (identical) twins

Monozygotic means 'coming from one egg'. These twins are formed when an ovum fertilised with one sperm splits in two and each half implants in the lining of the uterus and develops into separate babies. These twins have exactly the same genes and are therefore the same sex and look as alike as 'two peas in a pod'. The developing babies usually share the same placenta, which has two umbilical cords coming from it.

Dizygotic (non-identical)

These twins come from two separate ova and two different sperm. It sometimes happens that two or more ova are ripened at one time and each of them is fertilised and implanted in the uterus as two separate embryos. Each has its own placenta, they can be of different sex, and their genes are only as similar as those of any two siblings might be.

Twins may be born before their due date because two babies take up more room and together are heavier than one baby. They may need special care, depending on their birthweight and general health. Their parents certainly need extra help, and this would be arranged before leaving hospital if it was not done before the birth. There is a national Multiple Births Association with branches in all the States and Territories. If possible, parents should be told about the activities of this organisation, as there is a lot of exchanging of ideas about ways of coping, social activities, as well as the sharing of prams, pushers and other expensive equipment needed for twins.

Infants in child care

The care routines and needs of infants and older children in child care are integrated into the topics throughout this book. In Chapter 1, the challenges of caring for several infants with the current staff:children ratio were mentioned. Growth patterns are described in Chapter 4, care routines are discussed in Chapter 6 and nutritional needs in Chapter 7.

It must be emphasised that providing care routines for babies is not just the provision of physical care. Care routines enhance all other areas of development: social, emotional, cognitive, language. Everything a caregiver does for an infant should be a potential learning experience. Adult-infant interaction is a wonderful way for babies to learn. Adults learn lots too!

The first 3 years of life are of crucial importance to brain development. Recent research has pointed out the importance of the infant's experiences in helping or hindering brain development. This places huge responsibilities on caregivers and parents and reinforces the need for a partnership. The young infant needs consistency between home and child care. So it is vital that caregivers and parents talk together about the infant's routine, her likes and dislikes at home, so that the child-care centre can match these as much as possible (this is discussed in more detail in Chapter 6).

Research in Australia and the United States has shown that infants in childcare need:

- close, intimate relationships;
- continuity of relationships;
- health and safety;
- connections with family;
- educated caregivers who are knowledgeable and responsive (Lally 1998).

Relationships are important throughout life, but especially in infancy. This is the time when the infant learns to closely relate to another person, when trust is learned, where a smile and a gurgle are responded to with delight from both baby and adult. Intimacy between caregiver and infants can be lost in large groups. Let's compare the following two situations:

Think about walking into a babies' room of a large child-care centre. There may be 12 babies (or more) under 15 months of age with four caregivers. The room is large and the younger babies are lying or sitting supported on the floor; others are crawling and exploring, or taking those staggering steps that come when first walking. The caregivers are on the floor chatting and interacting with whichever baby is nearby. The toys are shared by all children.

The second situation is the same room with the same babies and staff. Here the large room has been set up with portable dividers that are sturdy enough for the crawlers to pull themselves up on, but low enough for staff to see over. Each staff member has three or four babies in his/her area and interacts solely with these children. The toys are shared by only four children.

The babies may well get as much attention from adults in both groups. The second group setting, however, could provide more intimate attention. Interacting consistently with the same person would help set up the intimate relationships that babies need, and also provide continuity of relationships. Health and safety is easier to achieve with a small number of babies. The risk of infection is less with small groups, as is the risk of toddlers tripping over younger babies on the floor. Caregivers are also able to form closer relationships with parents and other members of the babies' families.

There does, of course need to be some creative administrative planning to ensure that continuity of staff can be ensured over rostered days off, in-service, sick leave and annual leave. Some child-care centres have solved this problem to a certain extent by having permanent relief staff who get to know all the babies. While not ideal, this solution is much better than having total strangers with the babies.

Learning activities

1. Discuss pregnancy and antenatal care with a family who has recently had a baby. It will need to be someone who feels comfortable about talking with you. You will need to ensure confidentiality.
2. Do you think women (and their families) are able to find out enough about what happens during pregnancy and childbirth? Find out about childbirth education classes in your area.
3. Obtain some literature from the Australian Nursing Mothers' Association.
4. Observe an infants' room at a long-day care centre. Discuss the organisation of the group with the Group Leader or Director.

References

Barker DJP. (1994). *Mothers, babies and disease in later life*. London, BMJ Publishing Group.

Bower C, Stanley FJ, Nicol DJ. (1993). Maternal folate status and the risk for neural tube defects: The role of dietary folate. *Ann NY Acad Sci*, 678: 146–155.

Henderson-Smart D, Ponsonby A-L, Murphy E. (1998). Reducing the risk of sudden infant death syndrome (SIDS): A review of the scientific literature. *Journal of Paediatrics and Child Health*, 34(3):213–219.

Hoy W. et al. (1997). A health profile of adults in a Northern Territory Aboriginal community with an emphasis on preventable morbidities. *Aust NZ Journal Public Health*, 21 (2):121–126.

Kitzinger S. (1997). *Pregnancy and childbirth*. Sydney, Doubleday/Dorling Kindersley.

Lally R. (1998). Presentation: Healthy child care in Australia Conference, Melbourne, November.

NHMRC (1997). *The health effects of passive smoking*. Canberra, AGPS.

Roberts KA. (1995). A comparison of chilled cabbage leaves and chilled gelpaks in reducing breast engorgement. *J Hum Lactation*, 11(1):17–20.

Sheridan M. (1993). *From birth to five years: Children's developmental progress.* Melbourne, ACER.

Woodcock HC, Read AW, Bower C, Stanley FJ, Moore DJ. (1994). A matched cohort study of planned home and hospital births in Western Australia 1981–1987. *Midwifery* 10(3):125–135.

Further reading

Bruce T, Meggitt C. (1996). *Child care and education.* London, Hodder and Stoughton (especially Chapter 3: Work with babies: Physical development and care).

Greenman J, Sonehouse A. (1997). *Prime times: A handbook for excellence in infant and toddler programs.* Sydney, Addison Wesley Longman.

CHAPTER 4

The growing and developing child

HUMAN GROWTH AND development are ongoing throughout life. Although each individual is unique, there are many common needs. At all stages of human growth and development there is a need for food, shelter, exercise, a clean and safe environment, and the recognition of social and psychological needs.

A knowledge of how the human body works is helpful when thinking of how growth occurs. We have already discussed how the body systems are all developed within the first 12–16 weeks of pregnancy. Each system has its own structure and function and works with many other systems to ensure the stability and wellbeing of the whole body.

Skeletal system

Structure and function

The skeletal system is made up of many bones of different sizes and shapes (Figure 4.1). The main functions of this system are to:

- keep the body upright;
- protect vital organs;
- make red and white blood cells in the bone marrow.

The bones

- *The skull,* which protects the brain. It is made of several curved bones, which are not joined at birth to allow space for the fast brain growth that occurs in the first 2 years of life. The curved bones join

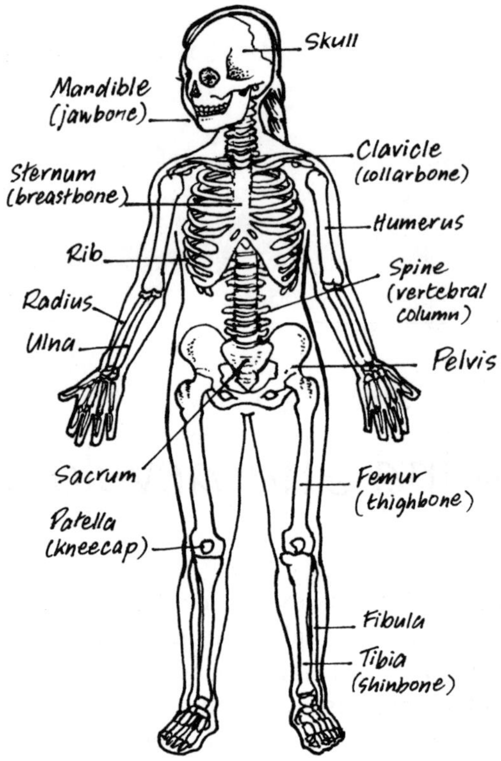

Figure 4.1 The skeletal system

up as the fontanelles close. The skull also contains the bony sockets for the eyes and the fine bones that make up the nose and nasal passages and sinuses. The maxilla (cheek bone) and mandible (jaw bone) are part of the skull and facial bones.

- *The vertebral column (spine)*, which is made up of vertebrae with discs of cartilage (soft bone) between each vertebra. These discs allow movement such as bending and also cushion each vertebra against jolts and jarring. The vertebrae are small at the neck and get bigger as they get down to the lumbar (bottom of the back) area. The vertebral column protects the spinal cord, which carries nerves to all parts of the body.
- *The sacrum and coccyx* are bones at the very base of the vertebral column. The sacrum is made up of fused vertebrae and the coccyx is similar to a little tail bone.
- *Two clavicles (collar bones)* sit at the front of the body, one each side of the sternum (breast bone).

- *The sternum* is a flat bone to which most of the ribs are attached.
- *The ribs* form a cage around the heart and lungs. There are muscles between each rib which assist the rib cage to expand while breathing.
- *The pelvic girdle* comes from the base of the spine and surrounds the lower part of the trunk. The front of the pelvic girdle meets closely with a piece of cartilage at the join. This piece of cartilage and other cartilage around the pelvis softens during labour so that there is more room for the baby to be born. The pelvic girdle protects the lower abdominal organs.
- *The two shoulder blades (scapulae)* sit each side of the top of the trunk and link the upper arms to the body.
- *The upper arm bone (humerus)* goes from the scapula to the elbow in each arm.
- *The lower arm bones (radius and ulna)* in each arm link the elbow to the wrist.
- *The wrist bones (carpals)* are attached to the *hand bones (metacarpals)*, which are joined to the *fingers (phalanges)*.
- *The femur* in the top of each leg goes from the hip joint to the *kneecap (patella)*.
- *The tibia and fibula* are the two bones in the lower half of each leg.
- *The ankle bones (tarsals)* are attached to the *foot bones (metatarsals)*, which are joined to the *toes (phalanges)*.

The joints

There are several types of joints that are needed to allow the bones and the body to move:

- Ball and socket joints such as the shoulder and hip.
- Hinge joints such as the knee, fingers and jaw.
- Pivot joints, as in the ankle and wrist.

Cartilage

This is softer and less rigid tissue than bone and is found in the external ear, the end of the nose, between the vertebrae and in the knee joint.

Growth plates

Children's bones have growth centres and growth plates, which allow continued growth and are not fully fused with the hard bone until after adolescence.

Muscles, ligaments and tendons

These are all made of soft tissue and are part of the musculoskeletal system. The ligaments are fibrous tissue which hold the bones together in order to prevent dislocation. Muscles and tendons are flexible and elastic and act to produce movement at the joints. These joint movements can be produced by small muscles (fine movements, such as those moving eyes and fingers) or large muscles (gross movements such as those moving arms and legs).

Muscle tissue is also found in the body where there is no bone but where movement and stretching is needed. Some of these muscles can be found in the heart, uterus and digestive system.

Development of motor skills

Babies

From birth, babies need to have opportunities to move muscles without the restrictions of clothing or bedding. Placing the baby on a waterproof covering without a nappy on allows the baby to kick and use large muscles. The room temperature should be such that the baby does not lose heat while uncovered. A safe space on the floor is a good place for babies to be able to roll. Some babies and parents might prefer light and loose clothing be worn.

Rattles to grab and to finger can be strung out over cots and prams and give lots of fine and gross motor experiences.

As motor development increases and the baby starts sitting and crawling, there should be plenty of safe, uninterrupted space to explore and lots of suitable toys to look at, to feel and to suck.

Talking about body parts also assists the baby to become aware of her own body. A baby learns during the first few months that her hands she looks at and the toes she sucks are part of her body.

Songs such as: *This little pig went to market* and *Round and round the garden,* which use body parts in the actions, are enjoyable, too (see *Merrily merrily songbook*).

Toddlers (12 months to 2½ years of age)

Toddlers need lots of room to push and pull wheeled toys, and lots of equipment to stack in and out of trolleys and prams. Safe climbing and rolling opportunities assist with gross motor development. Toddlers' motor co-ordination is still developing so they need uncluttered spaces in which to run.

Action songs about the body parts and bones continue to provide valuable learning experiences. Some examples are: *Head, shoulders, knees and toes* and *I wiggle* and *Open, shut them* (see *Merrily merrily songbook*).

Pre-school children (3–5 year-olds)
The pre-school child has much more control over his body movements and his balance. He enjoys riding a tricycle, getting around obstacle courses and having challenging climbing experiences. His fine motor skills are becoming increasingly developed, so lots of manipulative equipment with which he can build complex structures makes for useful physical and cognitive activity.

Other learning experiences about bones and muscles can include borrowing a skeleton from a science department of a local secondary school or a school of nursing and health sciences.

Songs are still enjoyed, and they now will refer to more detailed parts of the body such as left and right hands and feet as happens in *Here we go looby loo* (See *Merrily, merrily songbook*).

School-aged children
School-aged children need lots of exercise and this often comes in the form of more structured sports and games as the child gets older. Physical education programs are not only about competitive sport but can include walking, gardening and other related activities.

As children are able to read more fluently, they will enjoy books about the body if they are made easily available. There are also many commercial CD ROM programs about the body that are produced for children and are now available for use on computers.

Teeth

Teeth are needed so that food can be chewed and broken down into small pieces that can be swallowed easily. They are made from hard tissue and are covered with enamel. First teeth usually appear at about 8 months, though they can be as early as 4 months. There is enormous individual variation with teething, which is perfectly normal.

There are three main types of teeth (Figure 4.2):

- incisors, which are sharp cutting teeth situated in the front of the mouth;
- canines, which are pointed in shape and situated at the side of the mouth;
- molars, which are grooved and situated at the back of the mouth.

The first teeth to appear are usually the bottom central incisors, and then the top incisors. Children are teething almost continually from

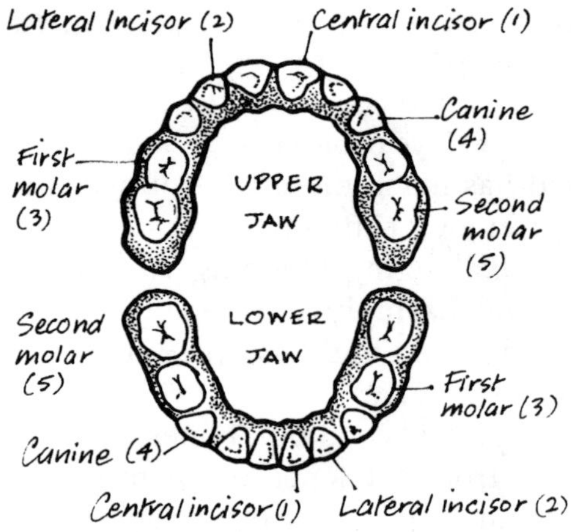

Figure 4.2 Teeth

when the first tooth appears until they have the second molars at the back of the mouth, which is usually when they are 2 or 3 years old.

The first dentition (baby teeth) start to fall out at 6–8 years and are replaced by permanent teeth.

The skin

The skin is made up of two layers (Figure 4.3):

- The epidermis or top layer, which consists of cells that are being replaced all the time. Melanin, a substance that gives skin its colour, is also produced in this layer.
- The dermis is the lower layer and is thicker than the epidermis. Nerves, sweat glands, hair follicles and sebaceous glands are found in this layer.

The skin is a complex organ with many functions:

- To provide a barrier that will prevent germs entering the body.
- To help maintain body temperature by the secretion and evaporation of sweat and by the hairs on the skin trapping warm air.
- To excrete some water and waste material through sweat.
- To protect the body from harm through the nerves, which sense pain, temperature and touch.
- To help make vitamin D from the reaction of sunlight on molecules within the skin.

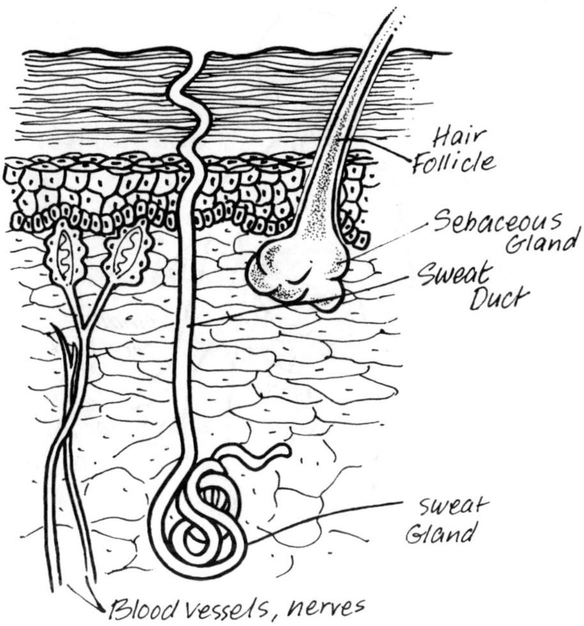

Figure 4.3 Skin

The digestive system

Digestion is the process by which food is broken down to substances that can be absorbed into the blood stream (Figure 4.4).

There are two methods for breaking down food (digestion):

- mechanical, as in chewing and churning the food;
- chemical, where enzymes made by the body alter the state of the food.

The mouth

The food enters the mouth, where it is chewed into smaller particles by the teeth. Enzymes in the saliva also mix with the food and fluid and start chemical digestion by changing the food or fluid containing starch. By the time the solid food is swallowed it has formed a ball (bolus), which easily slips into the oesophagus.

The oesophagus

The oesophagus is the tube that links the mouth to the stomach. The walls of the oesophagus contain muscles that help push the food down into the stomach. This pushing movement is called peristalsis.

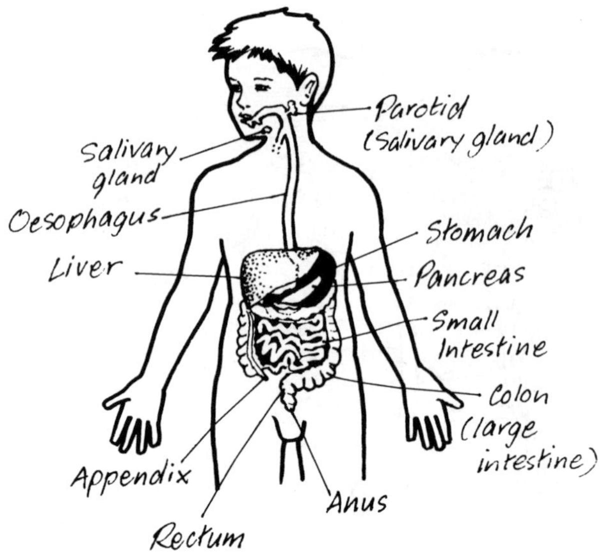

Figure 4.4 The digestive system

The stomach

The stomach has muscles (sphincters) at each end which close so that the food can be mixed and churned up with enzymes (gastric juices) and with hydrochloric acid, which are both secreted by the lining of the stomach. The gastric juices and hydrochloric acid continue the chemical breakdown of the food. In addition, the acid kills some of the germs that might have been on the food.

The small intestine

The food then enters the first part of the small intestine, which is called the duodenum. The duodenum has two tubes (ducts) entering it, one from the gall bladder and one from the pancreas. Bile, which is made in the liver and stored in the gall bladder, comes into the duodenum and helps with the digestion of fat. Enzymes from the pancreas also help with the digestion of fats as well as carbohydrates and protein.

The food is now almost digested and enters the rest of the small intestine, which is a very long tube. The walls of the small intestine contain many blood vessels and the digested food is absorbed as small molecules through the thin lining of the small intestine into the blood stream. The blood vessels then carry the food to the liver, which turns the food into substances that can be used by the body. This process is called metabolism.

The large intestine

The undigested material, such as fibrous food as well as water which remain in the small intestine, now pass into the large intestine. Here the water is reabsorbed into the blood stream and the undigested food is broken down by bacteria (*Escherichia coli*) into faeces. The faeces are excreted as waste material through the rectum and anus.

Respiratory and circulatory systems

Between them, the respiratory and circulatory systems play a major role in keeping the body working. The respiratory system (Figure 4.5) takes life-giving oxygen from the air breathed in and delivers it to the blood, which circulates through the body delivering oxygen and nutrients to tissues and cells. The blood also collects waste products in the form of carbon dioxide from food used up in the body cells and hands it over to the respiratory system, which gets rid of it in the air breathed out. As adults breathe in and out 15–20 times a minute (and children more frequently) these tireless activities of the respiratory and circulatory systems in exchanging oxygen and carbon dioxide in every cell of the body seem quite amazing.

The respiratory system

Upper respiratory tract

Air containing oxygen is breathed in through the air passages of the nose and goes through the pharynx (throat) and the larynx (voice box)

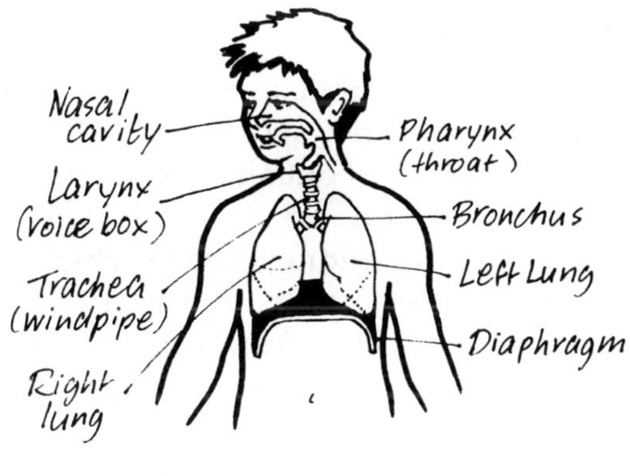

Figure 4.5 The respiratory system

at the back of the throat and into the trachea (wind pipe). The passages at the back of the throat are common to both the digestive and respiratory systems. It would be dangerous to get food into the trachea, so there is a structure (epiglottis) which protects the larynx from food entering when swallowing.

Trachea and bronchi

The trachea sits in front of the oesophagus and is kept open at all times by C-shaped rings of cartilage. The air goes down the trachea into the chest cavity. Here the trachea divides into two passages (bronchi), which again keep dividing into ever-smaller air passages in each lung.

Lungs

The lungs are spongy organs situated each side of the chest cavity. They fill with air when the large dome-shaped muscle (diaphragm) and the intercostal muscles (between the ribs) stretch and expand the size of the chest cavity.

Air sacs

At the end of the respiratory passages in both lungs are many air sacs (alveoli). These air sacs have very thin walls and are surrounded by very small blood vessels, which also have very thin walls. The oxygen from the air passes through the walls of the air sacs into the blood vessels.At the same time, carbon dioxide goes from the blood vessels into the air sacs; it then goes up through the structures of the respiratory system and is breathed out as a waste product. This process is known as the exchange of gases. The blood vessels containing oxygen merge into a large blood vessel called the pulmonary vein, which goes directly to the heart.

The circulatory system

Although the respiratory and circulatory systems work together, it is interesting to look at the circulatory system alone. Figure 4.6 shows how the main arteries and veins spread out all over the body and carry blood to and from the brain via the carotid artery and the jugular vein. The renal artery and vein go to the kidney, the brachial and femoral veins and arteries to the arms and legs. All body structures have a rich blood supply, which they need in order to keep functioning.

The heart

The heart is a very muscular organ that is undoubtedly the world's best pump. It beats approximately 72 times each minute in adults—that's 32 million times in a year—and is likely to keep working for at least 70 years. And to perform this incredible feat it needs its own blood supply just as any other tissue in the body. Heart attacks occur when the blood vessels supplying oxygen and nutrients to the heart become blocked and a small piece of heart tissue dies because of lack of oxygen. This causes the heart to stop working and then, of course, the rest of the body stops as well.

The major function of the heart is to pump blood into the major blood vessels so that food, chemicals and oxygen can be carried to tissues and cells in all parts of the body. The heart is divided into four chambers (ventricles and atria), which keep the blood containing oxygen from the lungs separate from the blood containing carbon dioxide coming from the rest of the body. Each of the chambers has a set of valves which prevent the blood from flowing backwards.

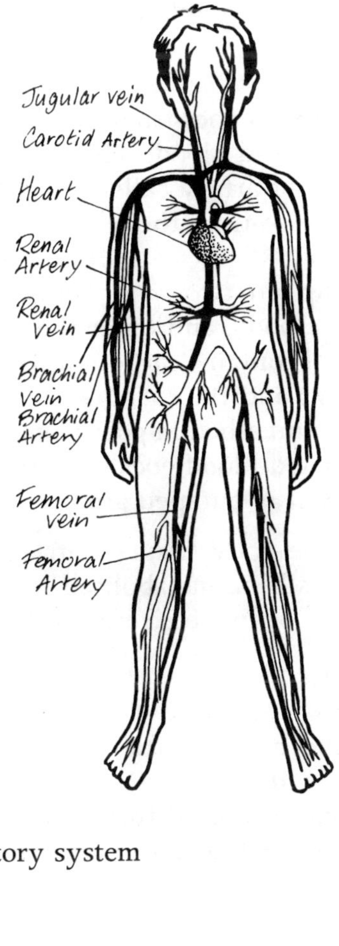

Figure 4.6 The circulatory system

Blood vessels

There are three main types of blood vessels:

- *Arteries* carry oxygenated blood to all parts of the body. There is one exception, the pulmonary artery, which carries de-oxygenated blood from the right side of the heart to the lungs.
- *Veins* carry de-oxygenated blood back to the heart, except for the pulmonary vein which carries oxygenated blood from the lungs to the left side of the heart. Veins have valves to help blood flow uphill from lower parts of the body such as the legs.
- *Capillaries* are very small blood vessels that form the link between the ends of the smallest arteries and the beginning of the smallest veins. The capillaries have very thin walls and deliver oxygen and nutrients to the tissue cells, while at the same time collecting carbon dioxide that the body does not want.

How the respiratory and circulatory systems work

- The large pulmonary vein goes from the lungs to the left side of the heart carrying oxygenated blood, which is then pumped out of the heart through the major artery called the aorta.
- Many large arteries arise from the aorta and go to tissues in all the parts of the body.
- The veins then join up into two major veins, one each from the upper and lower part of the body, and enter the right side of the heart.
- The blood (which still contains carbon dioxide) is then pumped from the heart to the lungs and the carbon dioxide is breathed out. The oxygen that has been breathed in goes from the lungs into the blood stream. This oxygenated blood goes back to the left ventricle of the heart and from there it is pumped around the body.

As well as carrying to the body tissues nutrients and essential chemicals from food, which has been metabolised in the liver, the blood also carries waste materials to be excreted by the skin and kidneys.

The blood

Blood carries around the body all the fluids and substances that are needed by the body cells. It is made up of both fluids and solids.

Plasma is a straw-coloured fluid that is mainly water but also contains essential substances such as antibodies, nutrients, chemicals and hormones, and clotting factor. The blood cells are suspended in the plasma. There are three types of cells:

1. Red blood cells (erythrocytes) are made in the bone marrow and are needed to carry oxygen around the body.
2. White blood cells (leucocytes) are made in the bone marrow and in lymph glands and help fight infection.
3. Platelets are made in the bone marrow and are needed to clot the blood if bleeding occurs.

The renal system

This is an excretory system, made up of (Figure 4.7):

- 2 kidneys, situated at the back of the abdomen near the waist
- 2 ureters
- a bladder
- a urethra

The kidneys act as a filter system for excess water and waste products that are carried in the blood. The blood goes to the kidneys through the renal arteries, where it is filtered through tiny structures called glomeruli. Excess water, waste salts and other materials are filtered off as urine, while the blood cells and other needed substances are saved to be recycled back into the blood and the circulatory system through the renal veins.

The urine passes down the ureters to the bladder, where it is stored until it is ready to be excreted from the body through the urethra. The male urethra comes out through the penis; the female urethra is in front of the vagina.

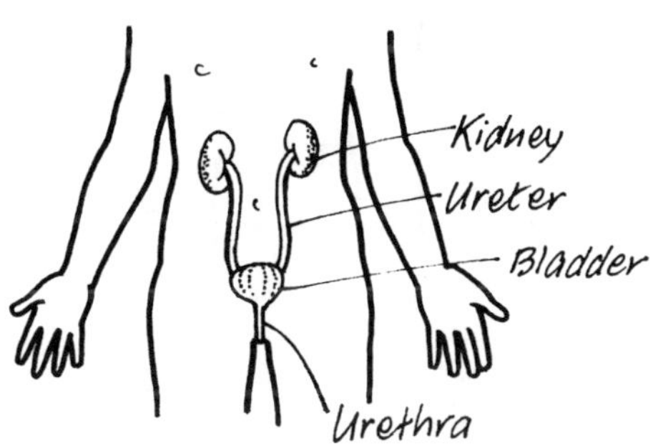

Figure 4.7 The renal system

The endocrine system

This is a system where chemical messengers (hormones) are made in glands in different parts of the body (Figure 4.8). The hormones are secreted directly into the blood stream and are necessary for the control and balance of specific body functions.

Pituitary gland

The pituitary gland, the controller of the system, is found at the base of the brain and secretes several hormones that stimulate the activity of other endocrine glands in the system. Growth hormone, which is needed to ensure growth in children, is also produced by the pituitary gland. If too little hormone is produced, the bones do not grow and the child is very short for age. If too much is produced in adults, the flat bones grow very big and the affected person has a large head and hands.

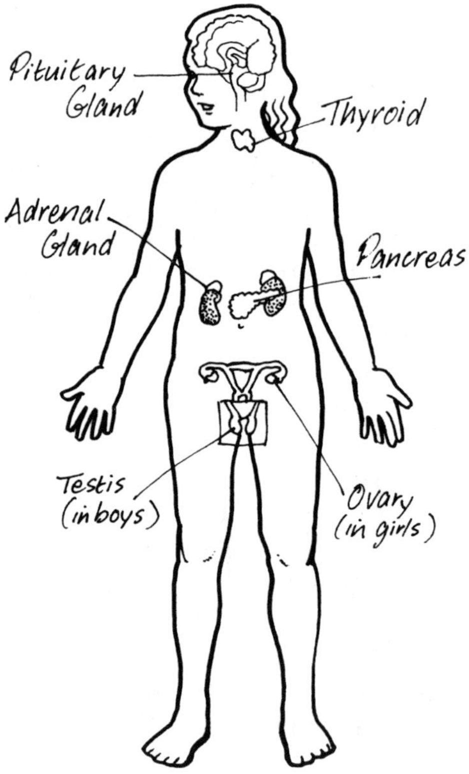

Figure 4.8 The endocrine system

Thyroid gland

This gland is situated in front of the voice box (larynx) in the neck and controls the metabolic rate (activity level) of the body. An over-active thyroid gland leads to over-active body functions where, for instance, the heart beats too fast and metabolising of food is too quick. Conversely, an under-active thyroid gland leads to under-active body functions. An unhealthy thyroid gland due to inadequate iodine in the diet of children can lead to severe intellectual disability called cretinism. This is rare in Australia and would be found at birth with the Guthrie test.

Parathyroid glands

These glands sit next to the thyroid and help to control the calcium, salt and water balance in the body.

Adrenal glands

The adrenal glands lie on top of each kidney and secrete several hormones, including adrenalin which helps the body cope with danger. Adrenalin is often known as the hormone of 'fright, flight and fight'. Other important hormones produced by the adrenal glands are androgens, which are male sex hormones and are generally found in a higher concentration in men, though women also secrete some androgens. Androgens can be made synthetically and are sometimes abused by athletes who want to build more muscle tissue.

Pancreas

There are patches of tissue in the pancreas which secrete the hormone insulin. Insulin is needed to control the metabolism of carbohydrate (sugar and starch) in the body. If little or no insulin is secreted, the body cannot metabolise the sugar and starch, and there are high levels of sugar in the urine and blood. This is the cause of childhood onset diabetes. Children who have diabetes will need to have injections of insulin and to monitor their food intake and blood sugar levels. We will discuss children with diabetes in Chapter 10.

Testes and ovaries

The reproductive organs are also endocrine glands and produce the hormones progesterone and oestrogen in females and testosterone in males. These hormones stimulate the development of the sexual characteristics of puberty and maintain the functioning of the reproductive system in adult life.

The nervous system

The nervous system (Figure 4.9) is one that relates to all parts of the body and its functioning. There are two main parts of the nervous system:

- The central nervous system, which consists of the brain and the spinal cord.
- The peripheral nervous system, which consists of nerves around the body.

Central nervous system

The brain is a complex organ made up of many parts. The two main parts are:

- The cerebrum, which is the largest part at the front, top and back of the brain. The cerebrum is responsible for the control of senses

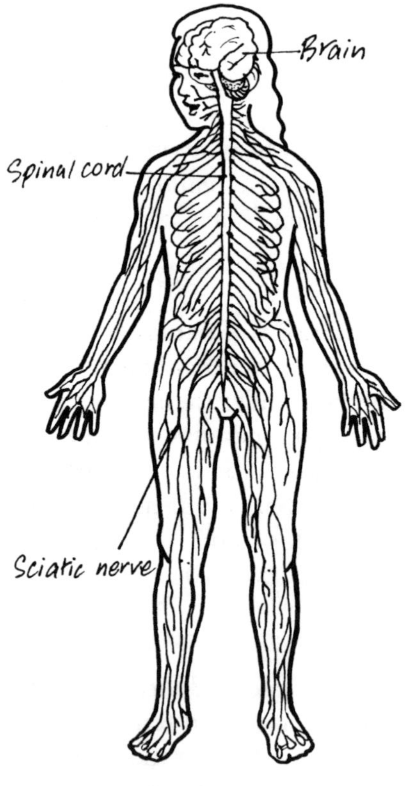

Figure 4.9 The nervous system

such as hearing and sight, voluntary movement, memory, learning, consciousness and many other cognitive functions. Other parts of the brain that are situated under the cerebrum control automatic functions such as heartbeat, breathing and movement of the digestive tract.

- The cerebellum is much smaller, and found at the bottom back part of the brain. It controls the co-ordination of body movements and balance.

The spinal cord

The spinal cord goes from the base of the brain to the lower back and is protected by the vertebrae in the spinal column. Nerves go out to all major organs of the body such as the heart, lungs and kidneys.

The brain and spinal cord are covered by layers of tissues called meninges. These layers contain cerebrospinal fluid, which nourishes and protects the brain.

Peripheral nervous system

Nerves arise from the spinal cord and go to outlying parts of the body, including the skin. Messages are sent to and from all parts of the body and the spinal cord. Some messages go to the brain for decoding. Reflex messages, such as occur when something hot is touched, go only to the spinal cord where the immediate reflex action of pulling the hand away from the heat is set into motion.

Nerves also tell us when something is wrong with any part of our body. Children experience pain when they fall and graze their skin. Ear infections cause pain and the child will cry and rub their ear, even when they are too young to be able to explain what they feel.

Child caregivers do much lifting in their work and need to take care that this is done in the correct manner. There have been many cases where lifting has caused back injury and the sciatic nerve has become painful.

The eye

The eye is protected by the bony eye socket of the skull, in which it sits (Figure 4.10). It consists of:

- Eyelids, which protect the eyes by blinking and shutting.
- A covering tissue called conjunctiva covers the eyeball. Dust and other unwanted substances are washed out by tears, which also keep the eye moist.

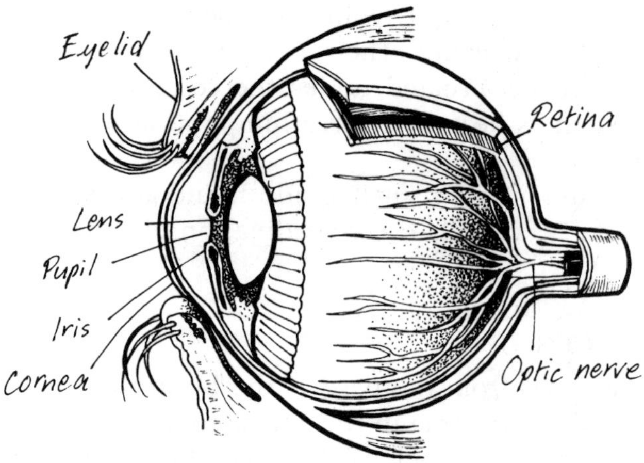

Figure 4.10 The eye

- The white of the eyeball is called the sclera and the clear part is the cornea.
- The iris is the coloured part of the eyeball surrounding the pupil (hole) that lets in or shuts out light.
- The lens is found behind the iris and is held in place by muscles that control the focusing mechanism to focus light on the retina which registers the image to the brain.
- The retina is on the inside lining of the eyeball and is made up of nerve tissue that is linked to the brain by the optic nerve. The image that comes into the eye through the pupil is picked up by the retina and transferred to the brain for interpretation This happens very, very quickly.

The ear

The ear is the organ of hearing and also plays an important part in assisting the balance of the body (Figure 4.11).

There are three parts of the ear:

1. The outer ear, which is made up of the flaps (pinna) on either side of the head. The pinna contain cartilage which keep the ear open so that sound can enter. The external ear canal goes down to the eardrum (tympanic membrane).
2. The middle ear is an air-filled cavity on the other side of the eardrum. The middle ear is connected to the back of the nose by the eustachian

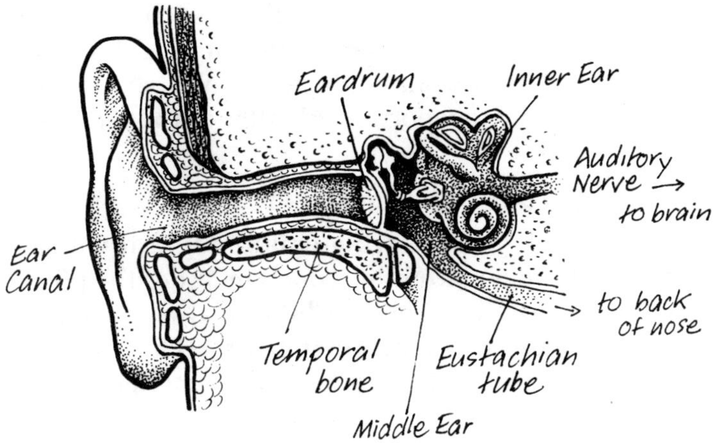

Figure 4.11 The ear

tube, which keeps the air pressure equal between this part of the ear and the outside air. Unequal pressure causes pain, which is sometimes experienced in a plane as it is coming down to land; in this situation a 'popping' sound can be heard as the pressure equalises. The middle ear also contains the smallest bones in the body, the hammer, stirrup and anvil, which transmit sound from the eardrum to the inner ear.

3. The inner ear contains the cochlea and other structures including the auditory nerve connecting the inner ear directly to the brain. The semicircular canals, which assist with body balance, are also found in this part of the ear.

How the ear works

Sound comes into the external ear and vibrates on the eardrum, which transfers the sound to the middle ear where it moves the three small bones so that the sound is amplified. The sound vibrations move into the inner ear, where the cochlea translates them into electrical impulses that are sent along the auditory nerve to the brain.

Ear infections are fairly frequent in early childhood, and this will be discussed in the section on middle ear infection in Chapter 5.

The defence system (or immune system)

This is a complex system that assists in resisting infection. There are more detailed examples of how the body defends itself against disease in

Chapter 5. Figure 4.12 shows the lymph glands such as the tonsils, adenoids, thymus, spleen and appendix and the lymph nodes, which enlarge during an infection. The lymphatic ducts are also shown. These ducts carry lymph, a fluid that transports antibodies to the blood stream.

Learning about the body

Professionals who work with growing children find it valuable to have an understanding of the whole child, which includes the physical structure and function of the child's body. Children also enjoy opportunities to develop an understanding of their own bodies. This requires a relaxed and open attitude toward setting up learning experiences and answering questions when children get to this stage of curiosity.

Toddlers learn about excretion from the digestive tract and urinary system as they develop the neurological (nervous system) competence

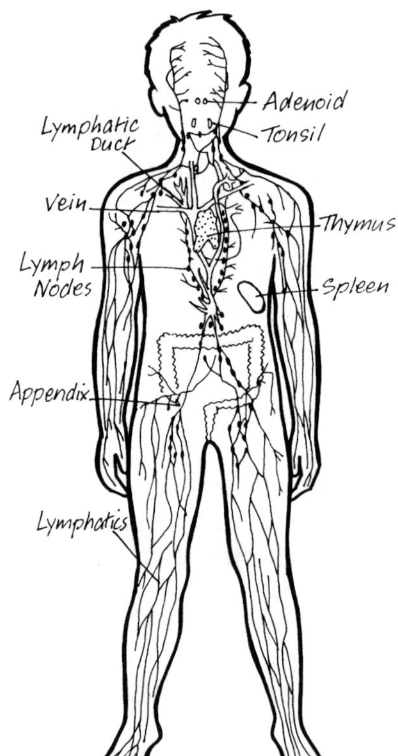

Figure 4.12 The defence system

that allows them to recognise the signals that precede defecation and urination. They are also very interested in the results, and may even wish to explore and touch their excreta. While touching should be discouraged, the child's curiosity should be respected and discussed. It is also an appropriate time to reinforce hygiene routines such as hand washing.

Dolls for toddlers to explore and to experiment with are useful in dramatic play activities and promote interest in bodies, as do stories and songs about bodies.

Older children whose conceptual development is more advanced often show a specific curiosity about how the body works and what they look like on the inside. Anatomical models can be borrowed for exploration and discussion. Special aprons that show internal organs are available commercially and can also be home-made. There are many books available which have cut-outs showing how the body works. Dramatic play opportunities that relate to health care can give useful opportunities for discussing body functions.

Bathroom language

Around 4–5 years of age children have much fun making up nonsense words and rhymes. This includes rhymes and words related to body functions, especially excretion; this can cause great hilarity among peers, though some adults find it difficult. It often happens at meal and other social times when the children are talking together. It is a very normal part of development and should be seen as such. Gentle guidance onto another interesting topic, while still valuing the language experimentation, is usually all that is needed to divert the conversation.

Exploring genitalia

Children will want to explore their own bodies, and this includes genitalia. Some adults find this disconcerting, though to a 2-year-old there is not much difference (if any) between touching his ear and touching his penis! It must be horribly confusing for young children to be encouraged by adults to sing songs about parts of their body and then find disapproval if a penis or vulva is touched.

However, children do need to learn what is acceptable in our society. Socially acceptable practices include learning to negotiate verbally rather than hitting or biting, sharing when possible, saying 'please' and 'thank you' at appropriate times, and all these practices are encouraged in child-care settings. Children whose stage of development allows them to understand these practices will also be able to understand that touching genitalia in public is not socially acceptable. At this period of development there is often a preference to go to the toilet privately, so the differences between private and public behaviour are becoming accepted.

Growth in the first 12 years

Growth patterns

Children grow at individual rates, but there are recognised patterns that are considered within normal limits The standard growth charts used in Australia show the wide range of body measurements that are considered normal for different ages (National Health and Medical Research Council 1981).

Ways of assessing the measurements

The charts shown in Figures 4.13, 4.14 and 4.15 are of weight height, and head circumference for females from birth to 5 years. The measurements for males are slightly larger in each category. Each chart has several curves for each measurement. These curves represent percentiles and are a way of recognising individual differences by comparing a child's weight, height and head circumference to the rest of the Australian population of that age.

Let us take height as an example. A child who is on the 97th percentile (top curve) of height for a certain age is taller than 97 percent of children at that age. A child who is on the 3rd percentile (bottom curve) is taller than only 3 percent of children at that age. Both children are seen to be within normal limits if their growth rates are consistent. They may also have very tall or very short parents. Very small babies will be assessed and observed carefully to ensure that there are no environmental reasons, such as sickness or inadequate nutrition, causing them to be so small.

The growth charts assist health professionals to note any untoward changes in the growth, or rate of growth, of a child and to make an early intervention that may avert any serious consequences. For instance, a sudden drop in weight gain is a real cause for concern and would trigger appropriate action to find the cause of the problem. A baby's head circumference is a gauge of how the brain is growing.

0–2 years

As can be seen by the growth charts, the first two years of life are a time of enormous growth. After that time the child's growth proceeds at a much slower pace.

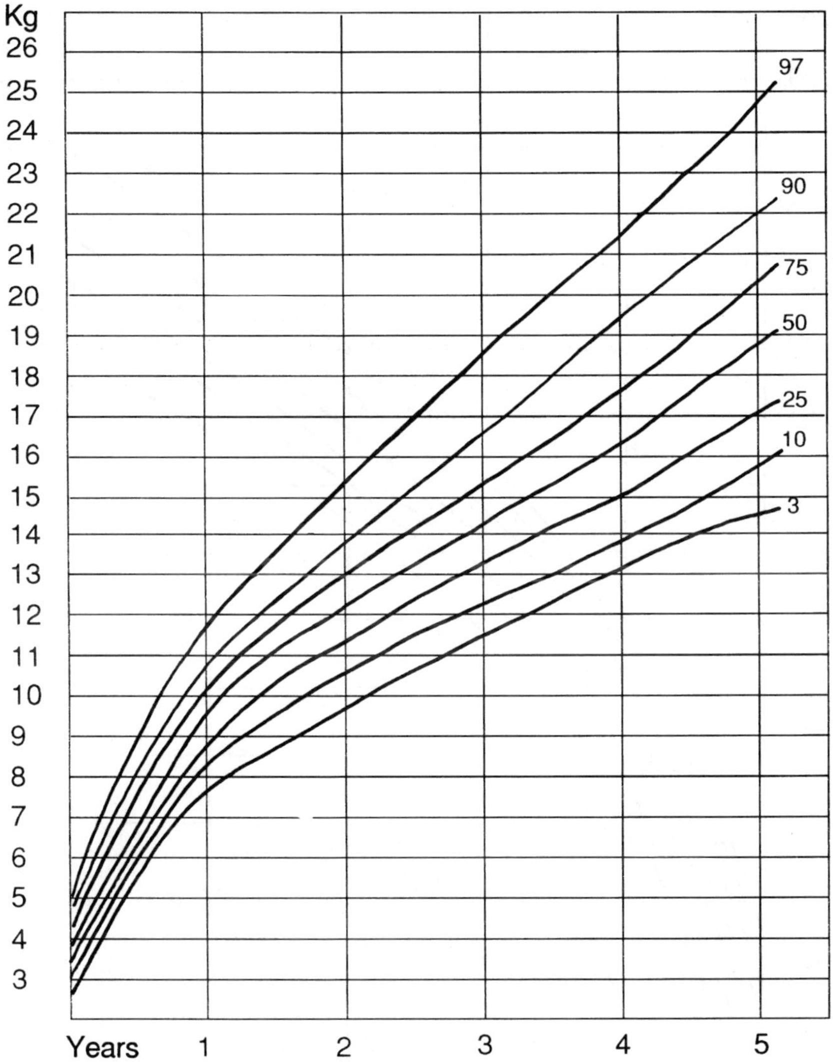

Figure 4.13 Girls' weight

Weight

Small babies whose parents are also small will probably gain weight more slowly overall than large babies whose parents are large. The weight gain of each baby should be consistent and incremental. Boys tend to be slightly larger than girls. The following growth rates are averages only.

- Babies gain weight rapidly in the first 5–6 months. After the initial weight loss immediately after birth, there is an increase of

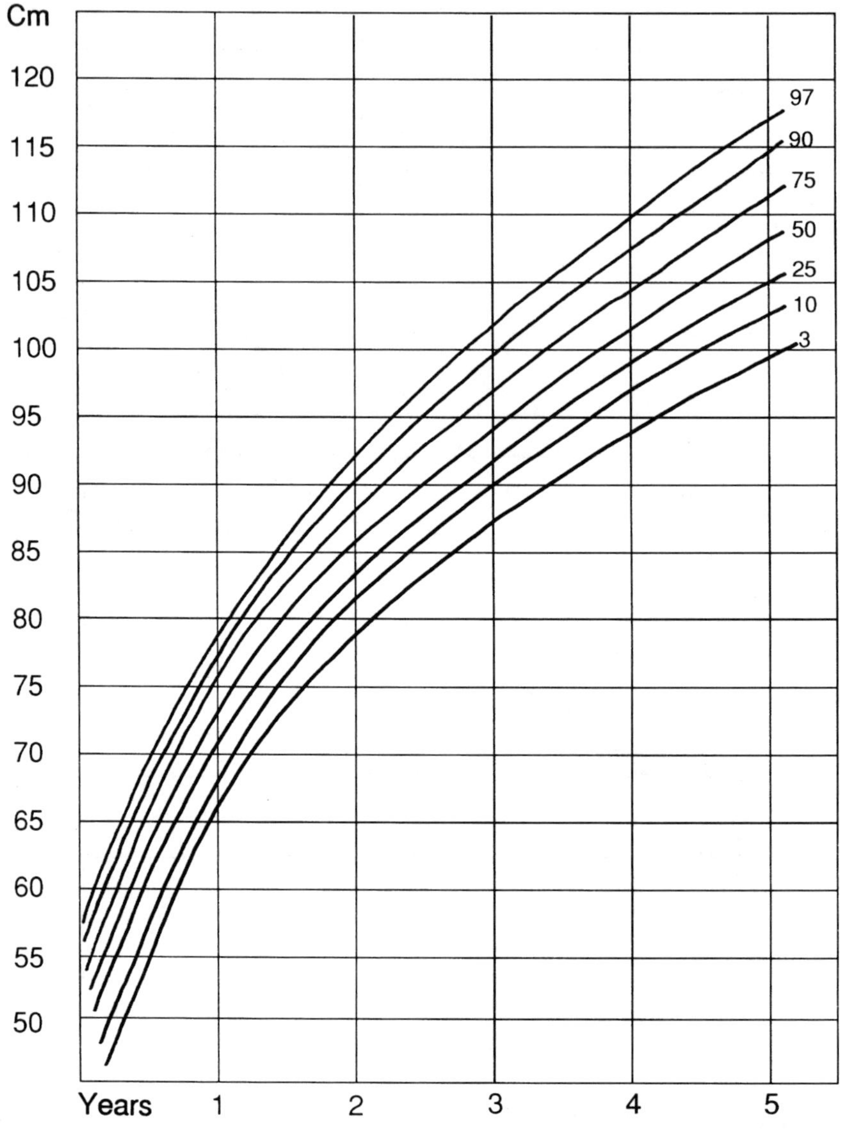

Figure 4.14 Girls' height

150–220g per week, which means that many babies double their birthweight by the time they are around 6 months of age.

- From 6–9 months the weight gain is slower, at about 90–150g each week.
- From 9–12 months the weight gain slows to 60–90g per week and by 12 months the baby weighs about three times her birthweight.

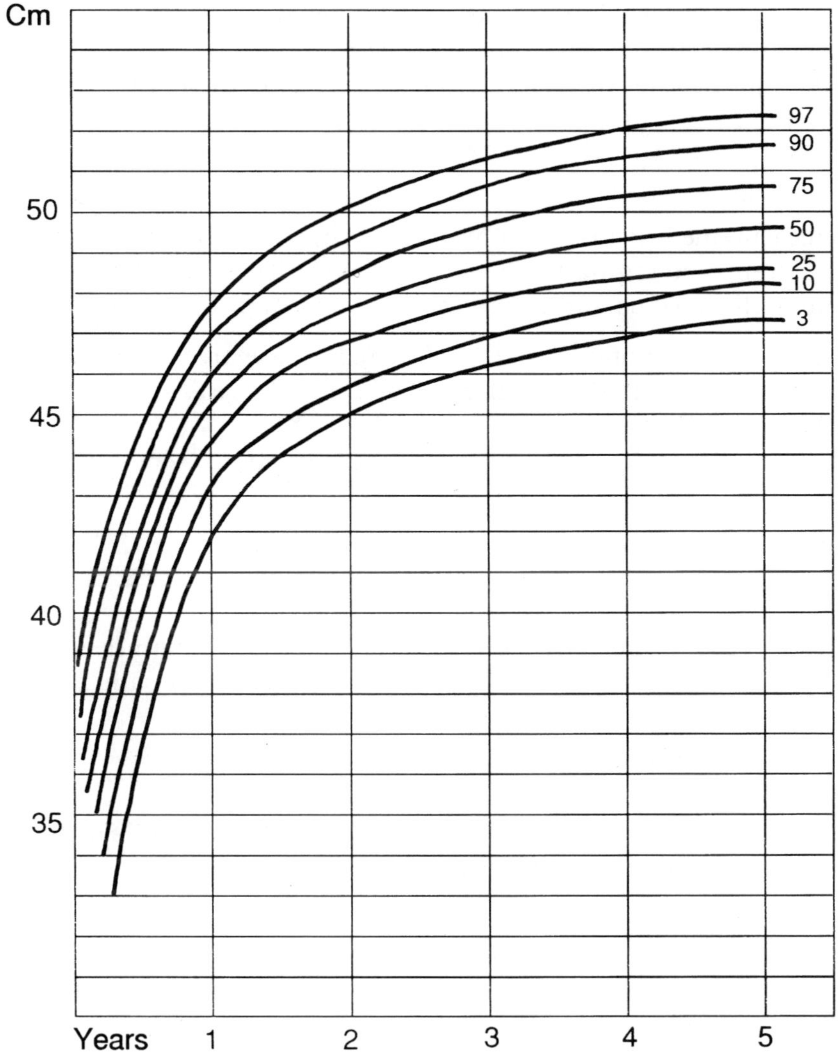

Figure 4.15 Girls' head circumference

- By 2 years of age the baby's weight is usually four times that of her birthweight.

Length (or height)

The individual differences of each baby also apply to length.

- There is an increase in length of about 13 cm in the 6 months after birth.

- The average length of babies at 12 months of age is around 75 cm, which is 20–25 cm more than at birth.
- The rate of growth slows in the second year to about 10 cm a year for the next 2 years.

Head circumference

This measurement is linked to brain growth, so it is important that head circumference be regularly checked. Growth that is too fast or too slow is potentially serious and needs to be investigated immediately.

- The head circumference at birth usually measures 32–36 cm.
- In the first year the head circumference increases by 10 cm, and reaches half its adult size.
- Growth slows down in the second year to about 3 cm a year.

2–5 years

Weight

There is a steady gain in weight over this period, though it is nowhere near as dramatic as in the first 2 years. The child will gain 2–3 kg per year.

Height

A child usually grows about 10 cm per year. At 3 years of age a child is about half their expected adult height.

Head circumference

The rate of growth of the head slows right down and is only about 1.25 cm per year for this age group.

5–12 years

This is a time when there is a steady gain in height and weight and a slower rate of head growth.

This situation changes dramatically in the later years of this period (an average of 11.5 years for girls and 12 for boys) when the pre-adolescent growth spurt occurs. These changes occur because of the secretion of oestrogen in girls and testosterone in boys. There is not only an increase in height and weight, but also in body shape. Emotions and feelings are also affected. Adult understanding and sensitivity is especially needed during this time.

Human development

Development is about growth and change. We all continue to develop throughout our lifespan, from adolescence to adulthood to middle and old age.

Child development concerns the changes that occur as the child moves from the total dependence of infancy to the increasing independence of being a toddler and pre-schooler to adolescence. Providing care and education for young children requires knowledge about how the child grows and changes within the social and cultural context of their environment.

Health and child development are closely related. However in this text we concentrate on physical health. Child development is a subject in its own right and is dealt with in greater depth in various other publications. Examples of such texts are given at the conclusion of this chapter.

Areas of development

Health depends on positive and ongoing changes in all areas of development, and not only in physical development.

- *Physical development* includes the physical health of the child and the growth parameters (height, weight, head circumference) discussed earlier in this chapter. The development of fine and gross motor skills is another aspect, as they refer to the way the child is moving and using all parts of her body. Hearing, vision and other sensory functions are also part of physical development.
- *Intellectual development* includes both language and cognitive skills such as reasoning, thinking and problem solving.
- *Emotional (psychological) development* means the ability to form effective relationships with other people who are close to the child.
- *Social development* involves the way the child learns to fit into the wider world, becoming able to care for herself and get along with others.

Emotional and social development are sometimes grouped together and referred to as psychosocial. Psychological health depends not only on emotional issues but also on the ability to form social relationships.

It is difficult to completely divide behaviours into separate areas of development because they are all very much intertwined. A baby who is reaching for a toy (gross, fine motor and cognitive) while smiling (social) at a trusted adult (emotional) and who then goos (language) and puts the toy in her mouth (sensory/cognitive) is performing an action in which all areas of development are involved.

How change occurs

There are many theories on how child development occurs. These theories are, of course, the proper study of special units in child development (there are many books available on this topic) but they are also relevant to health studies.

Social and cultural influences

Child development does not occur in isolation, but within the social situation of the family and the culture of the wider society.

Margaret Mead (1977), who studied families on Manus Island in Papua New Guinea, found that gross motor development and physical coordination of children was of the utmost importance because the community lived in houses over the water and the only transport was boats. Children need to be agile and to develop motor coordination skills at an early age in order to move around safely in this community.

Annette Hamilton's study (1981) indicates that the common milestones of gross motor development in Aboriginal children in remote Northern Territory communities may occur at an earlier age than happens with non-Aboriginal children in other settings.

Some cultures value the development of independence and self-help skills. Children are encouraged to dress and feed themselves from as early an age as possible. Other cultures emphasise the need for dependence, and to them it would seem neglectful if adults did not dress and feed children even up to school age.

Family size and the place within the family can also influence child development. An only child of a sole parent lives in a very different environment to the middle child in a family of five children where there are two parents and perhaps a grandparent living in the same house. Each situation has different strengths and potential problems, which may influence the individual child's characteristics and development.

Milestones

These are identified actions that signal a certain change within the continuing process of development. There is no exact age at which these milestones are achieved, but rather an age range in which they should happen. Each child is a unique individual and there are enormous developmental variations between children. Most children reach the milestones in the same order, but again there are individual differences; a few children start walking without ever having crawled.

Some of the actions that are milestones in the first 2 years are:

- *Gross motor development:* lifts head up, rolls over, sits without support, crawls, stands alone, walks, kicks ball . . .
- *Fine motor development:* eyes follow moving object, grasps rattle, reaches for object, builds a tower with four blocks . . .
- *Cognitive development:* repeats actions, recognises people, hunts for hidden objects, uses familiar objects such as a comb in the correct way, follows two directions . . .
- *Language development:* coos, laughs, turns towards a voice, imitates sounds, says mama/dada, combines two or three words . . .
- *Emotional and social development:* smiles at friendly faces, becomes shy with strangers, plays singing games such as pat-a-cake, starts to undress self . . .

Milestones form the basis for developmental assessment, which is an important part of health care. Health professionals, such as child-health nurses and paediatricians use milestones to help identify any potential developmental delay.

Child-care professionals use milestones in developmental checklists and charts as part of the process of keeping records of the development of each child. These records are necessary if the best care and educational programs are to be planned for individual children and groups of children. Developmental records are an essential requirement for accreditation of child-care centres (Principle 17, NCCAC 1993).

Health care

An important part of the health care of each child is the ongoing observation, surveillance, and assessment that should regularly occur from birth. These assessments happen on a regular basis at the child-health centre. Each State and Territory has its own facilities, which are free and available to all families in Australia. Community-health nurses, who are family- and child-health specialists, and other health professionals regularly assess the well child in order to keep the child well! Special baby health record books are given to families, and all health assessments noted. Immunisation records are also kept in this book. Sometimes there are milestone charts included in the back of the book and developmental advice for parents.

Observations

Observations of children are ongoing and involve many people. Parents need adequate information about what to expect at each developmental stage. Receptive community-health and child-care staff need to be available to discuss any concerns that parents might have. One of the important rules for child-health professionals is that the parents' observations and concerns are important and must be noted and respected.

Staff in children's services will observe children at all times, as this is part of the duty-of-care requirements. More formal observations should also be done, as these are another part of keeping health and developmental records and, again, are needed in order to plan a program of activities for each child. Each service will have a policy regarding regular written observations, which includes doing these more often when there is concern about a specific child.

Child screening and health surveillance

The aim of screening and surveillance is to identify children with needs who will benefit from early intervention.

In 1993 the National Health and Medical Research Council reviewed the policy and practices of health screening and surveillance for Australian children. The aim of these programs is to promote health and to prevent ill-health. The review committee looked at past and current practices in Australia and overseas and the economic viability of screening programs.

The following indicators of child health are monitored regularly in the first 5 years of life:

- height;
- weight;
- head circumference;
- hearing;
- vision;
- developmental progress;
- congenital heart disease (where the baby is born with some malformation of the heart or blood vessels;
- congenital dislocation of the hip (which will, if not treated early, prevent the child from walking with ease);
- undescended testes in boys (in the long term this can cause sterility);
- scoliosis (curved spine) in girls;

- immunisation;
- developmentally appropriate health promotion.

Developmental assessment and early intervention

There are many types of assessment tests in all areas of child development. These tests are carried out by health and education professionals who are trained in areas such as paediatrics, nursing, psychology, teaching, physiotherapy, speech pathology, occupational therapy and many others. Many of these people will be part of a special unit, often called an Early Intervention Unit (see allied health professionals in Chapter 12).

The aim of these assessments is to identify any areas of developmental delay and if possible find a cause that can lead to treatment. In all cases a program of activities will be implemented which aims to both reduce the level of developmental delay and try to prevent any potential long-term disabilities occurring because of this delay.

Child-care professionals are very much part of the program of activities. Sometimes special-education and child-health staff are employed part-time to work with individual children. These staff then assist the child-care professionals to continue the program on a regular basis.

Support for parents is an integral part of every program and child-care professionals are essential members of the team providing this support.

Needs of the child

All children have physical, social, emotional and intellectual needs. The fulfilment of these needs is the most important task for both parents and caregivers. Children are born with an inborn genetic potential that may not be realised if the environment is lacking in any way. Providing the best possible environment for children is of the utmost importance.

As mentioned in Chapter 3, there is current evidence based on work in the United States that brain growth in the important first year of life may be dependent on external stimulation from the environment. Babies who are in an environment that is intellectually stimulating are more likely to have a faster rate of brain growth than children whose environment offers little stimulation.

Physical needs

These are the basic needs of food, shelter, warmth and clothing, fresh air, activity and rest, and a safe environment. The best environment ensures that, in meeting these needs, the child's development and individual personality are taken into consideration.

Social needs

Growing children need to be part of a group. They need to develop the social skills of living with others, of valuing others and knowing they are valued themselves, so that feelings of self-respect are encouraged. Children also need to begin to learn the skill of self-care and independence within the context of stable social environments where there are familiar people and familiar routines and where there are opportunities to learn from experiences.

Emotional needs

Learning to give and return affection is a complex developmental experience. Much has been written on how this occurs in children. Bowlby (1953) was one of the first to emphasise the need for the development of attachment (bonding) with a primary caregiver, who was usually the mother, and the ill effects of not developing or of breaking these bonds. It is now generally thought that babies can form attachments with several people, but that these people need to have a consistent and intimate role in the life of the baby. This has implications for child-care staff when planning rosters and programs, as it is important to ensure that continuity of care and staff is as consistent as possible.

Intellectual needs

Babies need to be surrounded from birth by an environment that is rich in language and cognitive stimulation, and sensitive to the changing developmental needs of the growing child. There should be safe, yet challenging, places and things to explore and with which to experiment. There should be lots of opportunities to learn from experience and to problem-solve. Babies and young children thrive with lots of physical contact, talking, songs, rhymes and stories.

Some causes of identified special needs

Many children have a degree of developmental delay for which there is no obvious reason. Other children have a special condition that can be specifically diagnosed.

This topic is very important and there are many excellent texts available for caregivers (examples are cited at the end of the chapter). The aim of this short section is merely to give the physical background to the cause of a few of the more common conditions which are the reason for a child having identified special needs. The information contained here should be seen as providing the underpinning knowledge needed for a deeper understanding of these special needs.

Down syndrome

Down syndrome is a condition where, at conception, a chromosomal accident occurs. No one knows how this happens, though it occurs more often if the mother is over 40 years of age. Prenatal diagnostic testing for Down syndrome is offered to pregnant women over the age of 35 years.

Children with Down syndrome are born with recognisable physical signs. The eyes are slanted, the tongue large, and there are abnormal creases in the palms. The umbilical cord may be very short. Apart from the physical signs, the child will always have some degree of intellectual disability and will show developmental delay in many other areas.

Many children with Down syndrome attend mainstream children's services and schools, often to the delight of the staff and other children because of their affectionate and happy personality (if brought up in a happy environment). Extra assistance is often given with the young child who may need help with some physical activities in the early stages. Special education programs will also be set up to encourage cognitive development as much as possible.

Spina bifida

This condition is the result of a neural tube lesion where the external covering of the spine is not complete. This leaves the spinal cord exposed and unable to work. Spina bifida therefore causes physical disability which can be as severe as paraplegia. The degree of disability is linked to the size and site of the lesion. The lesion is most often surgically repaired at birth and would be treated like any other scar. The child with spina bifida may have no sensation in the limbs below the lesion. Care to prevent injury is needed here.

The degree of nerve damage may mean that the child may never be able to walk unaided and may need help with maintaining bladder and bowel function. There can be intellectual disability depending on whether the child also has hydrocephalus, which prevents the fluid around the brain from draining away.

Most children with spina bifida have no intellectual disability. The environment therefore needs to be arranged so that the child can become as independent as possible in a wheelchair or on crutches. Special assistance may be needed for toiletting.

Cerebral palsy

There are several types of cerebral palsy. In this condition, the central nervous system is not coordinated with the muscles. The cause is not always known, although sometimes birth injury is the cause; brain infection and trauma can also be causes. Often cerebral palsy is caused by something that happened before birth.

The severity of this condition is dependent on the muscles affected. Some children may have a lurching gait but be able to walk. Others will need walking aids or a wheelchair. Where the muscles of the face are affected, there will be great difficulty in talking and in communicating verbally. Eating and drinking will also be very difficult. The worst affected children will have no control over any muscles at all; they will not be able to sit unaided, talk, control their mouth movements or, in many cases, even smile.

One of the saddest problems with children who have the most severe forms of cerebral palsy is that it is very difficult to assess cognitive ability. Advances in technology have helped develop equipment—wheel-chairs for mobility and computers for communication—but such equipment requires some movement for successful use.

There have been many stories of adults who were thought to be profoundly intellectually disabled, who have found a way to communicate and have written about what it was like to be thought intellectually disabled.

Learning activities

1. Collect as many songs, rhymes and chants as you can that are about bodies and movement.
2. Discuss with others the ways you could plan activities that would encourage children to learn about their bodies.
3. Find out from whom you could borrow an anatomical model and skeleton.
4. Have a look at some catalogues for anatomical aprons. They are quite expensive, so think about how you might turn making one into a creative activity with the older children. You may need to do this over several weeks.
5. Visit your local Infant Health Centre (it may be called by a different name) and get a baby record book.
6. Find out how a child might be referred to the Early Intervention Unit.

References

Bowlby J. (1953). Child care and the growth of love. Harmondsworth, Penguin.

National Child Care Accreditation Council (1993). *Putting children first: Quality improvement and accreditation system handbook*. Sydney, NCAC.

Hamilton A. (1981). *Nature and nurture: Aboriginal child-rearing in North-Central Arnhem Land*. Canberra, Australian Institute of Aboriginal Studies.

Mead M. (1977). *Growing up in New Guinea*. Harmondsworth, Penguin.

NHMRC (1981). *Percentile charts*. Canberra, Australian Government Printing Service (AGPS).

NHMRC (1993). *Review of child health surveillance and screening*. Canberra, AGPS.

Further reading and resources

All song titles come from:

Nursing Mothers' Association of Australia. (1983). *Merrily, merrily songbook*. Melbourne, NMAA.

There is also a CD available with some of the songs included.

There are many other songs about body parts in other publications.

Body books for children

Brook JHR, ed. (1996). *My first book of the human body*. Collingwood, Ken Fin Books.

Dorling K. (1995). *My first body book*. London, HarperCollins.

Resources for caregiving staff

Freer M, Careen L. (1995). AECA Resource Book Series, Volume 2. *What do I look like on the inside*? Canberra, AECA. There is a video of the same title.

British Broadcasting Commission. (1998). *The human body*. Video Series.

Child development

There are examples of a Child Skills Checklist in:

Beatty JL. (1990). *Observing development of the young child*. New York, Merrill.

Faragher J, MacNaughton G. (1990). *Working with young children*. Melbourne, TAFE Publications, Victoria (see table of sequence of development in Appendix I).

Sheridan M. (1988). *From birth to five years*. Melbourne, Australian College of Educational Research.

General child development

Charlesworth R. (1992). *Understanding child development*. New York, Delmar.

Faragher J, McLean J. (1983). *Children's stages of development: birth to $2\frac{1}{2}$ years*. Melbourne, TAFE Publications, Victoria.

Faragher J. (1985). *Children's development: 3 to 5 years*. Melbourne, TAFE Publications, Victoria.

Children with additional needs

Palmer A. (1998). *Young children with additional needs*. Australian Early Childhood Association Research in Practice Series, Vol 5: No 2.

Children with Additional Needs. *Australian Journal of Early Childhood*. Vol. 20, No 4, 1995.

SECTION 2

Child Health and Child Care

CHAPTER 5

Infectious diseases

HEALTH, AS WE discussed before, is a positive state of physical, social and emotional wellbeing and not just an absence of disease. It is, however, impossible to attain this state of wellbeing if disease is present. Thus the prevention of disease is a major responsibility of child-care and early-childhood professionals.

Having frequent episodes of even minor infections can be harmful to the all-round development of the child. A child who is not well will feel listless and disinclined to eat, which affects growth and general wellbeing. The listlessness hinders the involvement in activities and learning experiences and this means there is a chance of a degree of developmental delay that could lead to further long-term problems with the health of the child.

Some infections, such as otitis media (middle ear infection, which is discussed later in the chapter) may cause conductive hearing loss during the course of the infection. This hearing loss hinders both language and social development and makes it difficult for the child to learn.

The prevention of infectious (or communicable) diseases is especially important in child-care settings. The risk of these occurring is very high due to large numbers of infants and young children mixing together at a stage of life when they are least able to fight infection. A high rate of infections in child-care centres has been noted in many countries including Australia, and many health professionals are becoming increasingly concerned at the number of respiratory infections and the episodes of diarrhoeal disease in these settings. A 1999 study shows that improvements in infection control practices by staff in child-care centres reduces the incidence of diarrhoeal and respiratory infections (Roberts et al. 1999).

Causes of infectious diseases

Infectious diseases are caused by micro-organisms (germs) which are too small to be seen by the naked eye, and by parasites. The germs infect the body in many ways. Viruses get inside body cells and may destroy or damage the cells. Bacteria often put a toxin (poison) into the body cells. Parasites get into or onto the body to feed, causing damage to the tissues.

Tables 5.2 and 5.3 (under 'Immunisation' in this chapter) list specific infectious diseases and include incubation periods, ways the disease is spread, symptoms, treatment and exclusion information.

Micro-organisms

The main micro-organisms that cause disease are:

Viruses

Viruses are the smallest of the micro-organisms. Antibiotics do not work against viruses, though some anti-viral agents are now being developed. Some of the diseases caused by viruses are:

- colds, influenza and other respiratory tract infections, middle ear infection;
- cold sores (herpes simplex) and other types of herpes, warts;
- erythema infectiosum (fifth disease), roseola (sixth disease);
- gastroenteritis;
- viral meningitis;
- chickenpox, measles, rubella, mumps;
- hepatitis A, B and C, Acquired Immune Deficiency Syndrome (AIDS).

Bacteria

Bacteria are larger than viruses, and antibiotics may be used to fight bacterial infections. There are many types of bacteria, which need different types of antibiotics. Chlamydia is a bacterium that acts rather like a virus and causes respiratory infection, trachoma (eye infection) and pelvic inflammatory disease.

Other diseases caused by bacteria are:

- middle ear infection;
- impetigo (school sores);
- whooping cough;

- haemophilis influenzae type B (Hib);
- diphtheria;
- tetanus;
- salmonella, shigella, gastroenteritis;
- meningitis;
- syphilis, gonorrhoea.

Fungi
The main diseases caused by fungi are thrush, tinea and ringworm.

Parasites
The main parasites are:

– protozoa, eg. giardia, which causes giardiasis;
– malarial parasite, transmitted by mosquitoes;
– metazoa, eg. worms, which cause a variety of internal diseases;
– mites, eg. scabies and head lice, which can cause skin infections.

Not all micro-organisms are harmful or cause disease. Some are very useful to the body and only cause harm when they get into the wrong place. For instance, the *Escherichia coli (E. coli)* bacteria in our bowel are necessary in this part of the digestive system, but dangerous if they contaminate food or get into the mouth or urinary system.

Cross-infection

Cross-infection is the term used when an infection goes from one person to another. The spread of infection happens in many ways, and some micro-organisms can be spread in more than one way. One of the aims in children's services is to prevent cross-infection.

Ways infection is spread

Many micro-organisms flourish in warm, damp, dark environments. They can live outside the body in the soil, in the air, on surfaces such as table tops in child-care centres, in food, on dirty hands or equipment, on toys. Given the right environment, bacteria multiply every 20 minutes or so, which means they grow into millions very quickly.

Conditions that hinder the growth of micro-organisms are extremes of heat and cold, strong sunlight and chemicals such as bleach and some other disinfectants.

Droplet or airborne (aerosol) spread and infectious discharges
Germs are spread when an infected person coughs, sneezes or breathes over another person. This also includes kissing. The germs are breathed into the warm dampness of the body, where they immediately start mul-

tiplying. Infants and young children sucking shared toys also contribute to this type of cross-infection.

Nasal and other discharges such as those from eyes, ears and throat are also very infectious. This means that infectious diseases are likely to be spread if noses are not wiped frequently.

Discharges from the nose, throat, ears and eyes can also dry up and be spread in the air to be breathed in by other children, staff, parents and anyone else in the child-care setting, thus transmitting the infection.

Diseases spread by this route include:

- all respiratory tract infections;
- measles, mumps, rubella, chickenpox;
- bacterial and viral meningitis;
- fifth and sixth disease;
- whooping cough;
- streptococcal throat infections;
- diphtheria;
- Hib.

Skin contact

Some infections are spread when the skin of the infected person comes into contact with the skin of another person. Cross-infection can also

Petro is 3½ years old and has a slight cold and runny nose. He is not really sick enough to be kept home from child care and is enjoying a collage activity at a table with a small group of other children. The caregiver does not notice his runny nose and Petro, who is very busy with his pasting, wipes his nose on the arm of his jumper. He also coughs a couple of times over the table and wipes his mouth with his hand, which he then puts back onto his collage and onto the table.

The micro-organisms that have caused Petro's cold are now all over the room and are being breathed in by all the other children. This could have been prevented by observing Petro more closely and making sure there were tissues available so that his nose could be wiped in an hygienic way and hands washed afterwards. At 3½ years of age, Petro would also understand simple instructions of turning his head to cough. He could have tissues nearby for him to use as a cover over his mouth.

Petro's illness may be mild and not serious to him, but another child could become seriously ill from complications of the same infection.

occur when the skin comes into contact with contaminated surfaces such as table tops, toys, dress-up clothes and hats.

Diseases spread in this way are:

- infectious skin sores such as impetigo (school sores) and cold sores;
- infestations of scabies and lice;
- ringworm and chickenpox from contact with the lesions.

It should be noted that chickenpox, which is a very infectious disease, is both airborne and transmitted by aerosol means as well as by contact with lesions.

Heng is 4 years old and enjoys dramatic play in the home corner. She is busy today getting ready to go shopping with her baby. She puts on a coat and then a hat before setting out. No-one remembered that Emily had been playing with the coat yesterday, even though she had a slight rash on her arm. Emily's mother rang today to say that the rash had become a sore, which has been diagnosed as impetigo. She is not coming back to the centre until treatment has been commenced and the sore will be covered with a waterproof dressing.

Heng is now at risk of also getting impetigo. This could have been prevented by encouraging Emily to play with other equipment until the cause of the rash was known. The dress-up clothes should also have been immediately washed when it was realised that Emily has impetigo.

Faecal-oral

This is one of the very common ways infection is spread in child-care centres where there are young children. Hands become contaminated with faecal matter (which may be such a small amount it is not seen), which is then spread to everything the child touches and to other children who touch the same objects. The hands of these children are now contaminated and the infection can easily get into the mouth. Some of the most frequent places where faecal contamination can be found are on toilet flush handles, taps, table tops, toys and nappy changing areas. Diseases caused by faecal-oral contamination are:

- all diarrhoeal diseases;
- giardia;

- hepatitis A;
- salmonella;
- shigella (dysentery);
- hand, foot and mouth disease;
- poliomyelitis.

Richard is just over 2 years old and very understandably wants to be independent. This includes going to the toilet, which he has just learnt to do. He climbs onto the toilet to defecate and is insistent that he wipe his own bottom, which requires much manipulative skill and so he cannot help getting some faeces on his hands. Richard flushes the toilet before he goes to wash his hands. He turns on the tap and runs his hands under the water very quickly without using soap. The caregiver is giving attention to another child while Richard washes his hands, so she doesn't notice that he has not done it properly.

Richard then runs back to the small blocks he was playing with before and builds a tower. Some of the blocks he has touched are picked up by Helena, who is crawling, and she immediately puts them in her mouth.

When morning tea comes a staff member says that Richard has washed his hands just before, so he is allowed to go straight to the table and picks up a piece of apple. He is also learning that it is fun to share, so he hands a piece of apple to Erica.

By now Richard has contaminated the toilet flush handle, the bathroom tap, the push button switch on the hand dryer, the bathroom door handle, the blocks that Helena put into her mouth, the table he was working on, the chair he sat on, the food he ate himself and that given to Erica, as well as his clothes and lots of other surfaces and articles!

Many children are now at risk of diarrhoeal disease which could have been prevented by better supervision of Richard's hand washing and by wiping the toilet flush button and the wash basin tap with a bleach solution after use.

Blood and body secretions

Some diseases are spread by blood-to-blood contact and with body secretions getting into the blood stream through a crack in the skin. Although this is not a common way of spreading disease in child care, extreme caution needs to be taken. General precautionary measures to prevent cross-infection will be discussed later. Diseases spread by blood and body secretions include:

- Hepatitis B and C;
- Acquired Immune Deficiency Syndrome (AIDS).

Maria, one of the caregivers in the babies' room, takes Jeremy to have his nappy changed. She doesn't realise that there are no gloves left until she has Jeremy on the table and she doesn't want to take him down, so decides to change the nappy without gloves. Jeremy is a well and happy baby but he has hepatitis B, though no one knows this. He has been a little constipated and has cracked some of the skin around his anus as he defaecated. There is consequently some blood in his faeces, though it is not at all obvious. Maria has been gardening at the weekend and has some small abrasions on her hands.

There is a real danger in this situation that blood from Jeremy's faeces may come into contact with the abrasions on Maria's hands and put her at risk of contacting hepatitis B, which could have been prevented by wearing gloves while changing the nappy.

Urine
Very few diseases are spread by urine, though contamination with urine can spread mumps and cytomegalovirus.

Body defences against disease

The body is not totally defenceless against invading germs. There are many in-built defence systems that help prevent infection getting into the body and fight the infection if it gets in.

Skin

Unbroken skin is a barrier to infection getting into the body by this route. The sebaceous glands in the skin also secrete sebum, which helps keep our skin from drying out and also contains an antiseptic that kills some germs. If the skin is broken through a cut or graze, then germs will be able to get in. It is important that child-care professionals, who need to wash their hands many, many times during the day, try to prevent their hands from becoming dry and cracked, which then provides an entry site for germs. Frequent use of hand lotion will help prevent this.

Body secretions

Some parts of the body, such as the eyes and lining of the nose, have a different type of skin cover. The skin cover in these places is fragile and extra protection is needed.

Tears, which contain a mild antiseptic substance, will start to flow if germs (or any foreign material such as dust) get into the eye. The tears help wash away the germs. The nose also waters if germs are getting in.

Mucus is produced in the respiratory tract in order to trap germs and dust. Saliva in the mouth contains a substance that destroys some germs, as does the hydrochloric acid produced by the stomach.

There is also mild antiseptic in semen, and the vagina and urethra secrete mucus to help trap germs.

Cilia

Cilia are fine hairs that line the top part of the respiratory system. These hairs collect dust and germs trapped by the mucus and irritate the throat, so that a person coughs to get rid of the infectious material. Smoking tends to poison and deaden the action of the cilia, which makes smokers more prone to respiratory infections. The cilia in smokers may 'wake up' and start working overnight when the smoker is asleep (and therefore not smoking) and this leads to the 'smoker's cough' in the morning.

The immune system

Immunity is the body's ability to fight infection. This happens in many ways (see Defence system Figure 4.12 in Chapter 4).

The body contains areas of lymphatic tissue such as the adenoids, tonsils, thymus, spleen, appendix and bone marrow. There are also many lymph nodes situated in the neck, under the arms, in the groin and throughout the abdomen. Lymphatic tissue and bone marrow make white blood cells, the body's vital 'defence forces' against germs. The white blood cells circulate in the blood stream and lymph vessels, constantly on patrol against invading micro-organisms which they will then attempt to destroy. People with leukaemia have a low white blood cell count; so do those who suffer from AIDS, which is why they are prey to the many opportunistic infections that beset them.

When there is an infection in the body, the 'defence forces' need reinforcements, so the lymph nodes swell up and make many more white blood cells to join the fight. The swollen lymph nodes also help to trap germs and kill them.

So next time you have a throat infection and the lymph nodes in your neck swell and are tender, you'll know there's a war going on in there.

Antibodies

Antibodies are specific substances produced by the lymphatic (immune) system to fight specific micro-organisms. The newborn baby already has some antibody protection from the mother. This protection is enhanced if the baby is breast fed, as antibodies are also secreted in the breast milk. This is called passive immunity as the antibodies are given directly to the baby from the mother and the baby does not have to make her own. For the first few months of life, maternal antibodies give the baby some, though not full, protection against the diseases to which the mother is immune.

Another form of immunity is where the body makes its own antibodies in response to meeting the infection.

Asha, aged 2, goes to a birthday party where she meets James, aged 3. James is a bit miserable that day and, unknown to everyone, he is getting the chickenpox. Chickenpox is spread through droplet infection in the early stages, so when James breathes on Asha he infects her with the chickenpox virus.

The chickenpox virus grows in Asha and her body tries to defend itself by making specific antibodies against the virus. However, Asha's immune system is still young and it has had no practice up until now in making chickenpox antibodies. She has none of her mother's antibodies left to help her, so the chickenpox virus temporarily wins the fight and some ten days later Asha gets chickenpox.

Luckily chickenpox is usually not too serious and so Asha, after a few days of being miserable and itchy, recovers after her immune system has had enough time to get rid of the virus.

Two years later, when Asha is at pre-school, she plays with Henrietta who is, unknown to everyone, about to get chickenpox. Henrietta coughs over Asha and the virus enters her body, but this time things are different.

Asha now has chickenpox antibodies in her body from the time she had the disease. These antibodies are ready to kill any chickenpox virus they meet. In addition, Asha's body remembers how to make these specific antibodies as it has done this before.

This time Asha does not get chickenpox, nor should she for the rest of her life. She has active immunity against chickenpox because she once had the disease.

Becoming immune by having the disease may be fine if the disease is not serious and there are no complications. However, graveyards are full of young children who died in earlier times from what are now preventable infectious diseases. Sadly, for these children the disease brought death rather than immunity.

Having infectious diseases a second time

There are many instances when people say they have had certain infectious diseases a second time. This can happen, but what is more likely is that one of the episodes may have been diagnosed wrongly, or the different episodes have been caused by similar but not identical germs. Children get a lot of non-specific rashes and these can be misdiagnosed as another disease, especially if there is an epidemic of that disease at that time.

Immunity from colds and influenza

People sometimes have colds or influenza from a viral infection, but having one attack does not confer permanent immunity. There are very many different kinds of cold and flu viruses and each attack is like getting a different disease.

Immunisation

Let us begin this section by establishing the fact that the terms 'immunisation' and 'vaccination' mean the same thing.

The number of children who died from whooping cough, diphtheria, tetanus, polio and other infectious diseases was very high until immunisation became more easily available. Deaths and permanent disabilities occurred from measles, mumps and haemophilus influenzae type B until quite recently, when vaccines against these diseases were developed.

Immunisation against rubella has almost eliminated the dangers of this virus to the developing fetus and the consequent disabilities it caused. It is interesting to note that it was an Australian, Norman Gregg, who first observed the link between rubella in the early stages of pregnancy and the birth of a disabled baby.

Immunisation confers active immunity without the dangers of having the disease. A small, controlled amount of the micro-organism (which is treated so that it is not harmful) or a substance that the body recognises as the micro-organism is injected or given orally to the child (or older person). This immunisation is enough to stimulate antibody production but not enough to infect the child and cause the disease. Babies may feel miserable for a few hours after immunisation. There may be a slight fever and red arm. Paracetomol, given strictly according to the manufacturer's instructions (on the side of the bottle), usually relieves these symptoms.

The antibodies made by the first immunisation dose may not be enough to confer adequate long-term immunity so that there may need to be a series of doses given over several months or years. Booster doses of tetanus and polio vaccine are needed throughout adult life, as antibody levels can fall.

Immunisation works in two ways:

1. It gives individual protection against a particular disease by antibody production and by boosting the body's ability to make the antibodies to that disease.
2. It gives community protection. The more immunised people there are within a community, the less likely it is that the disease can spread, because there are fewer people who can become infected and transmit disease to others. If immunisation rates are close to 100 percent, then the infection may not be able to spread at all and it will be eradicated from the population. An unimmunised older child in a child-care facility will put babies, who are not old enough to be fully immunised, at risk of getting preventable diseases.

Some years ago, the rate of full immunisation in Australia was less than 53 percent (Commonwealth Department of Health 1995) and the Commonwealth Government actively promoted ways to improve this. To this end, financial inducements were introduced. The full Maternity Allowance will not be paid until documentation of full immunisation status has been shown when the child has reached 2 years of age. Eligibility for Child Care Benefit payments are now also linked to evidence of full immunisation status for age.

A successful international immunisation campaign was carried out in the 1970s and 1980s against smallpox. High rates of immunisation were achieved and smallpox has now been eradicated from the world. It is hoped that polio will soon be eradicated, too.

History of immunisation

It is interesting that smallpox, which is now eradicated, was the disease that gave the first clues as to how immunisation works.

There was much infectious disease in England (and everywhere else) in the 18th century and many people died from smallpox. Those who contracted the disease but did not die were left with very badly scarred faces.

There was one group of people who seemed to escape smallpox even if they nursed patients with the disease, and whose faces were smooth and unscarred. This group of people consisted of the women who milked cows.

The nursery rhyme:

Where are you going to my pretty maid?
I'm going a milking sir, she said.

refers to the pretty milkmaid, who obviously had not had smallpox as she has no scars on her face.

Edward Jenner was the first person to note that the milkmaids (and some other farm workers) did not get smallpox as often as other people in the general population. It was known that cows often had a disease called cowpox, which was similar to smallpox in humans but not nearly as serious.

What was happening was that the cowpox virus (though no-one knew about viruses at this time) was being transmitted from lesions on the cows' udders to the milkmaids' hands. The milkmaids probably had lots of cracks on their hands, and this allowed the cowpox virus to enter their bodies. The immune system recognised the cowpox virus and made antibodies and the milkmaids became immune to smallpox as well as to cowpox.

The current immunisation debate

Rate of infectious diseases

At a world-wide level, rates of infectious diseases are still very high. Three million children die each year from vaccine-preventable infectious diseases, including whooping cough, mumps and measles.

It is ironic that some of the current concerns in Australia about immunisation have come about because of the success of past immunisation programs. The fact that diseases such as tetanus, diphtheria and polio are scarcely ever seen in countries such as Australia means that many people are unaware of the dangers of these diseases. So people are now questioning whether immunisation is necessary. We have much better living standards now than people in Australia had in the past, or than people currently have in developing countries. There is no overcrowding in most Australian households and sanitation and safe water supplies are in place.

'Has the improvement in living standards, rather than immunisation, been the real reason for the reduction in infectious disease?' many people ask.

That the improvement in living conditions alone is not enough to prevent infectious diseases is shown by the fact that the rate of diseases such as whooping cough rises when children are not immunised against this disease.

The recent reduction in sickness and death of children from Haemophilis influenzae type B is another case where recently introduced immunisation has dramatically reduced the disease in situations where there is no corresponding change in living conditions.

Side effects of immunisation

The safety of immunisation is also under scrutiny, with questions being asked about possible side effects. It would be misleading to claim that there are no side effects to immunisation. Infants often have a mild fever and feel a little grumpy after immunisation. Serious side effects have been documented, though these are very rare. On balance, the side effects of immunisation cause much less harm than would be caused by the diseases that are prevented by immunisation. In our grandparents' time thousands of children were paralysed by polio (infantile paralysis) and many died. Following immunisation, polio has almost entirely disappeared from Australia.

Many parents have had concerns about the whooping cough (pertussis) vaccine. A new pertussis vaccine is now available which does not have the potential side effects of the old vaccine. The new vaccine is more expensive, although this should not be a real problem for developed countries. The new vaccine is now on the recommended immunisation schedule throughout Australia. Developing countries will find it difficult, if not impossible, to afford the new vaccine.

There are children who are extremely allergic to a variety of substances, or whose immune system is depressed due to an illness, or who are taking drugs that suppress the immune system. Medical advice would be taken in these situations and it may be recommended that these children should not be immunised, or perhaps be immunised in a hospital where severe reactions can be immediately treated.

It is important to acknowledge that the benefits of immunisation far, far outweigh the very, very small risk of side effects. Immunisation reduces and eliminates serious illness, disability and death from infectious diseases.

Alternative medicine

The use of alternative medicine and homeopathic remedies has also spilled over into the immunisation debate. While these remedies may be perfectly harmless, there is currently no evidence that they confer any protection against infectious diseases.

Immunisation schedule

The National Health and Medical Research Council (NHMRC) is the Commonwealth Government body set up to develop policies, guidelines and procedures on all health issues. The immunisation schedule (Table 5.1) is regularly updated so that Australian children are offered the best immunisation cover needed to prevent diseases. Immunisation is available to all children at no cost, though some parents may choose to have their child immunised at a private facility.

Immunisation and child-care staff

(See also Chapter 11)

Working with young children places staff at risk of contracting infectious diseases. It is important that all staff check that their immunisation status is complete before starting work in a children's service. Boosters of tetanus, diphtheria and polio should be kept up to date every 10 years.

It is recommended that staff be immunised against hepatitis A if they are working with children under 2 years of age, where nappy changing is one of the duties. Children who have hepatitis A generally remain well, with no signs and symptoms, but they are infectious.

All staff working in children's services should be screened for tuberculosis prior to employment. This usually means a skin test and a chest x-ray. It is recommended that staff returning from long periods overseas are screened before commencing work with children in Australia.

Child-care staff should also take advantage of the flu vaccines which are available each year (NHMRC 1997).

Immunisation and child care

All child-care facilities have a unique and important role to play in promoting and explaining immunisation. Leaflets giving any new information, and Health Department pamphlets, should be available for

Table 5.1. National Health and Medical Research Council Immunisation Schedule (2000)

Age	Immunisation
Birth	Hepatitis B vaccine
2 months	Hepatitis B/ Haemophilus influenzae type B (Hib) vaccine Diphtheria/ Pertussis/Tetanus vaccine Oral Polio vaccine
4 months	Hepatitis B/ Haemophilus influenzae type B (Hib) vaccine Diphtheria/ Pertussis/Tetanus vaccine Oral Polio vaccine
6 months	Diphtheria/ Pertussis/Tetanus vaccine Oral Polio vaccine
12 months	Measles/Mumps/Rubella vaccine Hepatitis B/ Haemophilus influenzae type B (Hib) vaccine
18 months	Diphtheria/ Pertussis/Tetanus vaccine
4 years	Diphtheria/ Pertussis/Tetanus vaccine Oral Polio vaccine Measles/Mumps/Rubella vaccine
Year 7 at school (11–12 years of age) One month later 6 months after 1st dose	Hepatitis B vaccine (1st dose) Hepatitis B vaccine (2nd dose) Hepatitis B vaccine (3rd dose) **Note:** These vaccinations are not necessary if the person has been previously fully immunised for Hepatitis B
Prior to leaving school (15–19 years of age)	Adult Diphtheria/Tetanus vaccine Oral Polio vaccine
Post-partum (after birth) for non-immune women	Measles/Mumps/Rubella vaccine
50 years	Adult Diphtheria/Tetanus vaccine
Over 50 years (Aboriginal and Torres Strait Islander people)	Pneumococcal vaccine (every 5 years) Influenza vaccine (every year)
Over 65 years	Pneumococcal vaccine (every 5 years) Influenza vaccine (every year)

parents and in-service programs held for staff. New staff should be inducted into the children's service and have the immunisation policy clearly explained. The video, *Calling the Shots*, can be useful for staff education.

Immunisation policy

There are as yet no national statutory regulations relating to immunisation for child-care facilities although financial benefits such as Child Care Benefit may be withdrawn. This means that it is essential that each service checks the regulations in their State or Territory. Each child-care facility also needs to develop its own policies and practices in conjunction with parents and health professionals. The policy should be explained to parents, who should also be shown or given a copy of the policy. An immunisation policy should:

- Explain the risk of infectious disease and the protection immunisation confers. Written material about this should be available for parents. Where possible, parent evenings could include talks about immunisation (and other health issues).
- Note and record the immunisation status of each individual child. Documentation of this status should be supplied. Children who are unable to be immunised for medical reasons should provide documented evidence of the reasons for this.
- Documented evidence of staff immunisation status should also be included.
- Note when next immunisations are due for children and staff.
- Give written information and verbal explanations to parents of unimmunised children that exclusion from the service may be necessary if there is a case of a vaccine-preventable disease within the service.

Assisting parents

It is very important for a children's service to have a procedure by which a reminder note is given to parents when the child's next immunisation is due. The use of computerised records can make this a relatively simple procedure.

There are many children whose immunisation is incomplete, not because parents are opposed to immunisation but because the parents simply forgot to get it done. Sensitivity to the many demands on parents who may both be working is important and all help should be given to assist them to have their children immunised. This help should include health facilities being available at hours that suit working parents.

Vaccine-preventable infectious diseases

All cases of vaccine-preventable diseases, as well as some other diseases, need to be reported to a local health authority. Directors of children's services should ascertain the procedure for notification in their area. Table 5.2 lists vaccine-preventable diseases; Table 5.3 lists infectious diseases for which there is currently no vaccine available.

Each table lists the diseases in alphabetical order and gives details of:

- type of micro-organism that causes the disease;
- length of incubation period;
- mode of transmission (way the disease is spread from one person to another);
- signs and symptoms;
- treatment;
- exclusion policies for children and contacts.

Terms relating to infectious diseases

Incubation period

This is the time between the germ entering the body and the person getting the first signs and symptoms of the disease. Incubation periods vary for each disease; some such as chickenpox have an incubation period of 10–21 days, others such as Acquired Immune Deficiency Syndrome (AIDS) may have an incubation period of several years, during which time the person is referred to as HIV positive.

Epidemic

This occurs when there are a lot of people with the disease in one area at one time. Epidemics come and go. You might hear parents say: 'The centre has chickenpox', which means there is an epidemic of chickenpox in the child-care centre. Epidemics can be world-wide (pandemic) or local.

Endemic

This situation exists when a country or an area has a disease all the time. Head lice are now endemic in many schools in Australia. Respiratory infections are endemic in many child-care centres.

Table 5.2. Vaccine-preventable diseases

Disease: Organism Incubation period	Mode of transmission	Symptoms and treatment	Child/staff with disease	Contacts
DIPHTHERIA Bacteria 2–6 days Is often fatal but rarely seen in Australia owing to immunisation	Droplet Infectious discharges from throat	High fever Sore throat Yellowish-white membrane at back of throat Antibiotic treatment given	Exclude until medical certificate of recovery is obtained following at least two negative throat swabs. The last swab must be taken at least 72 hours after completion of antibiotics	Exclude all family and household contacts until medical certificate obtained Contacts may also be treated
HAEMOPHILUS INFLUENZAE type B (Hib) Bacteria 2–4 days Can be fatal	Droplet Contact with respiratory secretions	Fever Vomiting Headache Irritability Neck stiffness Breathing may be difficult Meningitis can occur Antibiotic treatment in hospital is necessary	Exclude until child has completed antibiotic treatment and is completely well Medical certificate of recovery should be obtained	May need antibiotic treatment Unimmunised children need immediate immunisation
HEPATITIS A Virus 15–50 days May leave people with weakened liver though full recovery is usual	Faecal-oral Possibly contact with urine	Loss of appetite Nausea Abdominal pain Dark urine Pale faeces Jaundice—yellow skin and whites of eyes	Exclude until medical certificate of recovery is obtained. Must be excluded for at least 7 days after onset of jaundice	No exclusion

HEPATITIS B Virus 2–6 months Can cause chronic hepatitis and cancer or cirrhosis of the liver later in life	Blood, and also semen and other body fluids–mainly IV drug use and unprotected sex	Abdominal discomfort Loss of appetite Nausea Dark urine Pale faeces Jaundice May have no symptoms	No exclusion	No exclusion
MEASLES Virus 8–14 days Can be fatal because of complications	Droplet Discharges from nose and throat	Runny eyes and nose Red eyes Cough Fever White spots (Koplik) in mouth Splodgy rash	Exclude for at least 4 days after rash appears	Immunised contacts not excluded Unimmunised contacts excluded until 14 days after the last case showed the first signs of the rash Those children immunised within 72 hours of first contact with measles can return to centre or school Babies under 9 months may be given immunoglobulin within 6 days of contact
MUMPS Virus 14–18 days Can damage reproductive organs and cause sterility	Droplets	Fever Headache Swelling of salivary glands	Exclude for 9 days or until swelling goes down	No exclusion

Continued

Table 5.2. (*Continued*)

Disease: Organism Incubation period	Mode of transmission	Symptoms and treatment	Child/staff with disease	Contacts
POLIOMYELITIS Virus 7–14 days Can be fatal or cause permanent physical disability	Faecal-oral	May be fever and listlessness Often no symptoms until paralysis appears	Exclude for at least 14 days. Medical certificate of recovery needs to be obtained	No exclusion
RUBELLA (German measles) Virus 14–21 days Usually a mild disease but dangerous to fetus if contracted by mother in first trimester of pregnancy	Droplet Nose and throat secretions	Fever May have swollen glands behind the ear Mild rash	No exclusion	No exclusion Pregnant contacts should seek medical advice
TETANUS (lock jaw) Bacteria Death is common in unimmunised persons	The tetanus bacteria grows under the skin, where there is no oxygen. Puncture wounds from gardening or dog bites are common infection sites	Paralysis of the face and neck muscles. Patient goes into spasm with sudden noises	Is not infectious but infected person would be hospitalised because of the seriousness of the disease	No exclusion of contacts

	Neonatal tetatus from bacteria in cord site is frequent in developing countries			
TUBERCULOSIS (TB) Bacteria 4–12 weeks though can lie dormant for many years Can be fatal	Droplet Secretions such as sputum	Usually affects lungs Fever May be undetected until routine skin test done	Inactive TB is not infectious Consult with Health Department regarding exclusion Staff and children with active TB are excluded until treatment has been given for one month and after medical certificate is obtained	May need to have skin tests Health Department will advise
WHOOPING COUGH (pertussis) Bacteria A very serious illness in babies and young children. Can be fatal	Droplet Infectious discharges from nose and throat	Fever Running nose Severe bouts of coughing Vomiting after coughing	Exclude until totally well and until antibiotic treatment has been taken for at least the first 5 days of the 14 day course	Exclude unimmunised contacts under 7 years of age for 14 days after last contact with infection and until antibiotic treatment has been taken for at least the first 5 days of the 14 day course

Table 5.3. Infectious diseases for which there is currently no vaccine available

Disease: Organism: incubation period	Mode of transmission	Symptoms: treatment	Child/staff with disease	Contacts
CAMPYLOBACTER Bacteria 1–7 days	Faecal-oral Contaminated food or water	Diarrhoea, abdominal pain, fever May need antibiotics	Exclude until diarrhoea has ceased	Exclusion not required
CHICKENPOX (Varicella) Virus 10–21 days A vaccine is available but not yet approved for routine use Varicella virus can cause shingles (herpes zoster) in older people	Droplet Contact with lesions	Fever Runny nose Tiredness Very itchy rash which is like small blisters DO NOT give aspirin	Exclude until all blisters are dried Must be excluded for at least 5 days after rash appeared	Exclude children and staff who have immune deficiency or are on immunodepressant drugs such as treatmeant for leukaemia Pregnant women should seek medical advice
COLD SORES (Herpes simplex) Virus 3–10 days	Contact with lesion	Small blisters, often around mouth Virus stays in body, so cold sores recur Some anti-viral creams available to prevent sores	Keep staff or child away from babies under 2 months of age	Exclusion not required

COMMON COLD see: Respiratory infections.				
CONJUNCTIVITIS Bacteria and virus May be caused by allergy 1–3 days	Contact with eye secretions or discharge and contaminated objects	Redness of whites of eye/s Eye may have sticky discharge Antibiotic oitment/ drops may be given	Exclude until discharge from eye has stopped	Exclusion not required
CRYPTOSPORIDIOSIS Parasite 10 days	Faecal-oral May be transmitted from animals	Diarrhoea—may contain mucus Abdominal pain Loss of appetite Vomiting	Exclude until diarrhoea has ceased	Exclusion not required
CYTOMEGALOVIRUS Virus 3–12 weeks but not accurately known	Body fluids, including tears, saliva and urine	Often no symptoms May have sore throat and swollen lymph glands in neck No treatment	Exclusion not required	Exclusion not required Pregnant women should seek medical advice
DIARRHOEA Bacteria, viruses, parasites Variable incubation period	Faecal-oral	Frequent loose bowel actions May have vomiting and fever May have abdominal pain or cramps	Exclude until all symptoms cease May need to have faeces tested for organism before returning	Exclusion not required

Continued

Table 5.3. (*Continued*)

Disease: Organism: incubation period	Mode of transmission	Symptoms: treatment	Child/staff with disease	Contacts
depending on the organism causing the diarrhoea		Loss of appetite Antibiotics given for bacterial infection Treatment available for some parasitic infestations Glucose fluids given to replace body fluids lost through diarrhoea and vomiting		
ERYTHEMA INFECTIOSUM (Fifth disease or slapped cheek syndrome) Virus 1–2 weeks	Droplet Secretions from nose and throat	Mild disease Fever Red cheeks Itchy rash on body and limbs No treatment	Not excluded	Not excluded Pregnant women and persons with immune deficiency should consult doctor
GASTROENTERITIS see Diarrhoea				

GIARDIASIS Parasite 5–15 days	Faecal-oral	Some persons have no symptoms Drug treatment is usually given to kill parasite. Medical advice should be sought	Exclude until all symptoms cease May need to have faeces tested before returning	Exclusion not required
GLANDULAR FEVER (Infectious mononucleosis) Virus 5–7 weeks	Saliva	Tiredness Swollen glands Is confirmed by blood tests Not common in young children	Not excluded, though may feel very tired and need to stay home	No exclusion
HAND, FOOT AND MOUTH DISEASE Virus 3–7 days	Contact with fluid in blisters Through droplet spread and saliva Faecal-oral (virus is present in faeces for several weeks)	Fever Blisters in mouth, on hands and feet May feel generally unwell Sore mouth may hurt when eating No treatment—treat symptoms Seek medical advice if fever persists or child has headache	Exclude until blisters have dried	No exclusion

Continued

Table 5.3. *(Continued)*

Disease: Organism: incubation period	Mode of transmission	Symptoms: treatment	Child/staff with disease	Contacts
HEAD LICE (Pediculosis) Parasite 7–10 days	Contact with eggs or lice from another person's hair. Can be direct contact or sharing of hats, combs, bed clothes or other items	Itching on scalp Eggs can be seen sticking to hair Hatched lice crawl among the hair Hair should be treated with approved lotion and combed with fine tooth comb Bed linen and other items in contact with head should be washed	Exclude until treatment carried out	Check for signs of head lice and treat if necessary
HEPATITIS C Viral 6–8 weeks	As for Hepatitis B	As for Hepatitis B	No exclusion	No exclusion

HUMAN IMMUNO-DEFICIENCY VIRUS (HIV) Infection which causes acquired immuno-deficiency syndrome (AIDS) Very variable but often 2–12 years	As for Hepatitis B/C Can also be transmitted from mother to child *in utero* and through breast milk	May have flu-like illness at start of incubation period. Infectious throughout incubation period New treatment available, results still uncertain	No exclusion if healthy Should be excluded on medical advice if cases of chicken pox or measles in child-care setting	No exclusion
IMPETIGO (School sores) Bacteria 1–3 days	Contact with sore or discharge from sore through touch, clothes or bed linen	Moist sore on skin which is yellow, flat and crusty Must be treated with antibiotic cream or medicine	Exclude until treatment has commenced. All sores must be covered with waterproof dressing	No exclusion
INFLUENZA see: Respiratory infections				

Continued

Table 5.3. *(Continued)*

Disease: Organism: incubation period	Mode of transmission	Symptoms: treatment	Child/staff with disease	Contacts
MENINGITIS Bacteria or virus Less that 7 days	Droplet Discharges from nose and throat	Fever Vomiting Headache Stiff neck May become irritable and drowsy Bacterial meningitis is usually more serious than viral Diagnosed by lumbar puncture. Child may need hospitalisation Antibiotics given for bacterial meningitis	Exclude until completely well	No exclusion, but may need preventive antibiotics
MENINGOCOCCAL INFECTION Bacteria 3–4 days	Droplet Discharges from nose and throat	May cause meningitis or blood poisoning (septicaemia) Fever Vomiting Headache Irritability	Exclude until completely recovered Will need antibiotic to help prevent spread of infection	Not excluded May need antibiotics and/or immunisation

		Neck stiffness Fitting Will need antibiotic treatment in hospital		
Respiratory tract infections—upper (colds, influenza) Viral 1–3 days Can cause complications of croup and bronchitis See: Streptococcal throat infection	Droplet Nose and throat secretions	Fever Headache Sore throat Running nose and eyes Complications include infection going to the lower part of the respiratory tract with coughing which is bronchitis or pneumonia	Exclude if child is unwell	Not excluded
Ringworm Fungus Incubation period varies	Contact with lesion, clothes or other contaminated items Can be caught from animals	Flat ring-shaped lesion appears on skin. Can occur on all parts of the body Is treated with fungicide lotion	Exclude until treatment has commenced	Not excluded

Continued

Table 5.3. (*Continued*)

Disease: Organism: incubation period	Mode of transmission	Symptoms: treatment	Child/staff with disease	Contacts
ROTAVIRUS Virus 48 hours	See Diarrhoea May also be spread by nose and throat secretions	See Diarrhoea	See Diarrhoea	See Diarrhoea
SALMONELLA Bacteria 6 hours—3 days	See Diarrhoea Contaminated food also causes the disease	See Diarrhoea	See Diarrhoea	See Diarrhoea
SCABIES Parasite—mite 2–6 weeks if first infestation 1–4 days if re-infestation	Contact with skin Sometimes by contaminated articles	Mite burrows under skin, between fingers and toes and in skin folds Very itchy Needs to be diagnosed and then treated with appropriate lotion Care should be taken with the treatment of babies and pregnant women	Exclude until treatment has commenced	Not excluded, although should be checked for infestation
SCARLET FEVER Bacteria 1–7 days Very rarely seen Comes from same family of	Droplet	Fever Sore throat Vomiting Rash and red tongue Can lead to kidney disease	Exclude until antibiotics have been taken for 24 hours and the child feels well	No exclusion

bacteria as impetigo and streptococcol sore throat		Is treated with antibiotics		
ROSEOLA (SIXTH DISEASE) Virus 10 days	Droplet Nose and throat secretions	Fever Splodgy rash over body No treatment—is usually a mild illness	No exclusion	No exclusion
STREPTOCOCCAL SORE THROAT Bacteria 1–3 days	Droplet Secretions from nose and throat Contact with contaminated articles	Fever Sore throat Loss of appetite Swollen glands in neck Throat may be swabbed to identify micro-organism Treatment with penicillin or other antibiotics Can become very ill and have long-term complications such as heart and kidney disease if untreated	Exclude until treated and feels better	No exclusion

Continued

Table 5.3. (*Continued*)

Disease: Organism: incubation period	Mode of transmission	Symptoms: treatment	Child/staff with disease	Contacts
THRUSH (Candida) Fungus 2–5 days in babies	Contact with secretions from mouth Contact with contaminated articles Faecal-oral if infection in digestive tract	White sore spots in baby's mouth—makes feeding difficult May go through digestive system and cause rash around anal area Can infect other parts of the body—especially in adults Treated with fungicide drops or cream	No exclusion, but feeding utensils and toys should be kept separate	No exclusion
TOXOPLASMOSIS Parasite—protozoa Incubation period uncertain—may be from days to months	From cat's faeces From infected meat that is not cooked well enough	Often mild illness or without symptoms May have fever and generalised aches and pains Can damage sight Disease dangerous to fetus if contracted by pregnant women	No exclusion Pregnant women should seek medical advice	No exclusion

Specific infectious diseases

There are some diseases about which people working in children's services should have detailed information, such as otitis media, hepatitis B and C, and HIV/AIDS.

Otitis media

This is a common infection in childhood. Otitis media (middle ear infection) is not in itself infectious unless pus is discharging from a ruptured ear drum. However, the respiratory infection causing the middle ear complications is very infectious.

Otitis media occurs frequently among young children. It happens much less often in children who are cared for in their own home compared with children who attend family day care. The rate of otitis media among young children attending centre-based care is very high indeed (Skull et al. 1999). It is because it occurs so often in child-care centres that a detailed description has been included here.

In the past, the long-term seriousness of otitis media has been underestimated by health and child-care professionals. Parents are certainly concerned by the number of episodes of otitis media a child has; they also worry about the number of times their child needs to stay home from child care.

Otitis media is a not a life-threatening illness but it can have serious effects on language and social development, and on behaviour and learning.

How otitis media occurs

The structure of the ear was described in Chapter 4, where the diagram shows that the ear is divided into three parts: outer, inner and middle. The middle part of the ear is linked to the back of the nose by the eustachian tubes—one from each ear.

Young children, especially those in child-care centres, are frequently exposed to germs that cause infections in the upper part of the respiratory tract. These infections may only seem minor, but the germs can go from the back of the nose, up the eustachian tube (or tubes) to the middle ear. The middle ear is damp and dark, an ideal place for these germs to grow. The middle ear, which should normally only contain air, then becomes inflamed and fluid and pus start to form. The eustachian tube/s become swollen and the fluid is unable to drain away.

This fluid and pus fills the middle ear space. The eardrum is unable to vibrate properly, which means that sound cannot be conducted from the eardrum through the middle ear. Nor are the small bones able to vibrate. There are therefore not enough sound waves made to transmit to the inner ear and the brain. The child's hearing is thus impaired. This is called *conductive hearing loss*, which will be discussed later in this chapter.

The pus and fluid in the middle ear can build up to such a level that the ear drum bulges and can burst. Pus then runs out through the outer ear canal. This pus contains germs and should be treated as an infectious discharge.

The eardrum will heal once the infection has gone but there will always be some scar tissue, and the eardrum will be less flexible and less able to pick up sound waves. The damage done by the ruptured eardrum may cause some permanent hearing impairment, even if only slight.

Physical signs and symptoms

A child who has acute otitis media will frequently have a high temperature and feel very miserable. A baby may rub at the infected ear and cry, and an older child may say the ear hurts. Some children may show very few signs and symptoms, and so parents and caregivers do not realise that the child has otitis media.

A medical examination of the ear will show that the eardrum is inflamed and perhaps bulging, which confirms the child has otitis media.

Treatment

This depends on the organism causing the infection, though very few medical practitioners would try to isolate the germ from each child. In many cases the original cause is a viral infection which then becomes re-infected with bacteria. Consequently the child is often given antibiotics to treat the infection.

Signs of conductive hearing loss

There are many signs that may be the first indication that a child is, or has been, suffering from conductive hearing loss:

- Inattentive
- Unable to concentrate
- Easily distracted

- Seems not to hear, especially in large groups
- Has difficulty in pronouncing words or is slow with language
- Does not respond when his name is called.

These signs may not always be present, as conductive hearing loss fluctuates with the degree of infection and the amount of fluid and pus in the middle ear. Sometimes the child will hear well when there is no infection and at other times hear very poorly.

Testing for conductive hearing loss

Any child who shows signs of hearing loss at any time should have formal hearing tests. The tests done should include audiometry, which will test the hearing very exactly. There have been many recent advances in audiometry, so that the hearing of young children, including babies, can now be very accurately tested. These tests, which are quite painless, usually involve placing electrodes on the child's head and measuring how much the brain reacts to sound.

Conductive hearing loss and young children

The first 2 years of life are crucial for the acquisition of language. The child needs to be surrounded by language, by different sounds and tones, by stories and songs. A child who has even a slight degree of hearing loss is going to miss many of these sounds and will be unable to discriminate between the many tones that make up language. This child may then have some developmental delay in language acquisition, which can make learning more difficult. Socialisation may also be affected as the child gets older.

Role of the caregiver

There are many practical things that caregivers can do that will help the child with conductive hearing loss.

- Observe children carefully for signs of otitis media.
- Communicate closely with parents regarding the child's episodes of otitis media.
- Try to reduce room noise by having rubber stops on the legs of chairs and having some carpeted areas.
- Ensure that background noise is kept to a minimum, and this includes music.
- Have small-group work, where the child can hear easily away from the larger group.

Special notes

Conductive hearing loss

Many of the signs of conductive hearing loss could also apply to Attention Deficit Hyperactivity Disorder (ADHD), which will be discussed in Chapter 10. There is a risk of misdiagnosing a child, and hearing assessments should always be done before a diagnosis of ADHD is made.

Conductive and sensori-neural hearing loss

There are two main types of hearing loss and the difference between them should be noted.

- Conductive hearing loss occurs when the sound waves are not carried across the eardrum, through the middle ear. The main cause of this type of loss is otitis media.
- Sensori-neural hearing loss occurs when something is wrong with the structures in the inner ear, such as the cochlea or the auditory nerve. This can be caused by damage to the fetus during the development of the ear. Before immunisation, rubella during the early part of pregnancy used to be a major cause of sensori-neural hearing loss. Other causes can be infection such as meningitis. A degree of sensori-neural hearing loss occurs in old age. Environmental noises can also contribute to this type of hearing loss, thus there are occupational health regulations about the wearing of ear muffs in noisy industries. Adolescents may well be damaging their hearing by listening to very loud music, whether live, on the radio, stereo or through walkman headphones.

- Talk with the child on a one-to-one basis and have children do the same.
- Make sure the child can see your face when you talk. This may mean gently touching the child's arm to gain attention.

Amplification devices

The child with conductive hearing loss mostly does not wear a usual type of hearing aid. More common is an FM receiver worn by the caregiver, which is linked to headphones worn by the child. The caregiver's voice is amplified, which helps the child hear much more clearly.

Otitis media with effusion (glue ear)

Sometimes the child has so many infections that they never really clear up. This leads to the middle ear always being full of thick white fluid that is rather like glue. The child is generally well, though his hearing is always a concern.

The current treatment is to place a fine tube called a grommet into the middle ear through the eardrum. The grommet/s allow air into the middle ear and let the fluid drain away and they are kept in until the middle ear is clear of fluid.

There is always a danger the grommets may fall out, which is not a serious situation but should be noted in the child's record and the parents told when they collect the child. Care should be taken to keep the external canal of the ear dry and this may mean that the child will not be able to go swimming. A copy of the care protocol for each child should be kept at the child-care setting.

Aboriginal children and otitis media

In some Aboriginal communities, families may live in overcrowded housing where there are many young children. Respiratory infections are common and the rate of otitis media among these children is the highest in the world.

In the Northern Territory in some Aboriginal groups a high percentage of babies rupture at least one eardrum before they are 12 months old. The infections start as soon as they return home from hospital. Many babies had their hearing tested at birth and were found to have no hearing loss. Tested again some weeks later, the babies showed definite conductive hearing loss (Boswell et al. 1995).

It is interesting that often these babies do not show clinical signs or symptoms of the disease: that is, they do not appear sick or distressed.

Redness around the eardrum can be seen on examination with an otoscope and disease-causing micro-organisms can be grown from the secretions at the back of the nose.

Hearing loss, particularly from a very early age, can obviously cause problems with language development. The maintenance of culture is made more difficult if children cannot easily hear the stories the older people tell. It may be that in the child-care settings and classrooms of some Aboriginal communities, the majority of children will have a degree of conductive hearing loss at some time, and this could impair learning. It can be difficult for caregivers and teachers to identify which specific children have otitis media and are therefore at risk of conductive hearing loss.

Infectious diseases that are spread by blood and other body fluids: Hepatitis B, C and AIDS

We have already discussed how the spread of these diseases can be prevented in child care by effective measures for infection control. It is important, though, for child-care workers to have an understanding about these diseases so that they can give the best care to any infected children and also to protect their own health.

Hepatitis B

This is now vaccine-preventable and so should not occur though there is a relatively high incidence amongst immigrants. Hepatitis B immunisation is now recommended for all newborn babies and for adolescents in Australia.

Hepatitis C

The incidence of hepatitis C is on the rise because of the increasing use of injected drugs, and these trends are a major national concern.

Hepatitis C is much more infectious than AIDS. It is spread mainly through blood, though sexual transmission is possible. Drug users who share equipment are at high risk of getting hepatitis C. Children in child care might be infected by needle-stick injuries, so that checking the outdoor area and sandpit each morning is important (this is discussed in Chapter 8). Inadequate hygiene measures with toothbrushes could also be a potential cause of transmission in child care (see Chapter 6).

A person infected with hepatitis C may not have any symptoms and be unaware of having the disease. This means they may unknowingly transmit it to many others. As with AIDS, the infected person may remain well and not become seriously ill for many years. The cause of death from hepatitis C is mainly due to cirrhosis or cancer of the liver.

The Australian National Council on AIDS and Related Diseases has linked health education and prevention measures for hepatitis C to those used in the AIDS education programs. The ethical responsibilities of children's services toward a hepatitis C-infected staff member or child attending their service are similar to those described for HIV/AIDS.

Acquired Immune Deficiency Syndrome (AIDS)

This disease (like hepatitis C) often brings about an emotional response because of misinformation. It is described in detail here in order to dispel the myths and to discuss the ethical responsibilities of children's services.

Human Immune Deficiency Virus (HIV) infection and AIDS are not common among Australian children. It is important for caregivers to understand the disease so that they can give the best care to an infected child and also safeguard their own health.

AIDS is a relatively recently discovered disease. The first cases noted were in the United States in the early 1980s, where doctors observed an increase in young men dying of a rare form of cancer. This was baffling to the health profession as they did not know what was causing the deaths.

Slowly the information about AIDS was put together and this is what was found:

- AIDS is caused by a virus that has been named the Human Immune Deficiency Virus (HIV).
- The virus is spread from person to person by the exchange of blood, semen or other body fluids.
- The incubation period may be from 2 to 12 years or even longer.
- The disease probably originated in Africa.

Australia implemented HIV/AIDS education programs very early on. The development of the programs involved many representative groups—the gay community, intravenous drug users, sex industry workers, parents, community participants and health professionals. Special programs were set up by Aboriginal and Torres Islander people for their communities. The current number of HIV-positive people in Australia is about 18 000 (1 : 1000 of the total population) of whom most are men.

Many African countries have very high rates of HIV infection and in some places up to 30 percent of pregnant women tested are HIV positive. These countries do not have enough money to test all pregnant women or to implement wide-reaching health education programs, and so the number of cases is still very high.

HIV infection

The first signs that a person may be infected is a cold or flu-like illness that clears up and the person then appears quite well. They may continue to be well during the incubation period over several years. Without a blood test, a person will usually not know they are infected with HIV until the first signs and symptoms of AIDS appear.

Despite lack of symptoms, a person infected with HIV becomes infectious at the first contact with the virus, but this cannot be identified until the antibody level has risen enough to be measured. This is called the 'window' period and it is the time when an infected person could give blood without tests showing any infection, as happened in Victoria in 1999 when a child became infected with HIV after a blood transfusion. The donor in this case had only recently become infected and this did not show up on the blood test.

Persons who are infected with HIV without being sick are called carriers. All carriers appear to be infectious throughout the long incubation period. Any carrier can transmit the infection to others without knowing they are HIV positive.

An HIV carrier slowly develops signs and symptoms of acquired immune deficiency syndrome, which is the actual disease caused by HIV. Long-term exposure to the virus during the incubation period eventually causes the immune system to break down. Because of the immune deficiency, infections such as a cold, which were previously mild, now become serious illnesses. More and more infections occur, which lead to increasing disease, debility and, eventually, death.

Treatment

For people with HIV, it has been found that early treatment with antiviral agents can slow down the onset of AIDS itself, but it is too soon to say whether people can be completely cured. The treatment is complicated and the drugs are expensive and have many side effects. The success of treatment depends on people at risk of HIV infection being treated regularly so that treatment can be commenced immediately after the infection has been confirmed.

For people with AIDS it also important to treat the symptoms and provide the best possible care for the person. This care is emotional and spiritual as well as physical, and there are specialist units for AIDS patients at many large hospitals.

There is, as yet, no immunisation available to prevent AIDS though many scientists ae working on a possible vaccine.

Transmission of HIV

- Sexual penetration with an infected person of either sex means that the vaginal fluids or semen can enter the blood stream of the uninfected person. Sexual activity often causes small cracks in the lining of the vagina or anus (in the case of anal intercourse). These cracks are enough for the virus to enter the blood stream. Cracks are very likely to occur in the lining of the anus because it is quite fragile. This is why the first cases of AIDS in America were found in men who were practising homosexuals.
- Sharing syringes for intravenous drug use also means sharing blood. When a needle is put into a vein, a little blood flows back into the needle and the end of the syringe. This blood then mixes with the substance being injected into the next person. If four people are sharing a needle, the last person will get a small amount of each of the other three people's blood.
- Blood crosses over the placenta at birth through the umbilical cord between mother and baby. A mother who is HIV positive may infect the baby at this time.
- HIV may also be secreted in the breast milk and infect a baby in this way.
- In the past many boys and young men with haemophilia were infected through routine blood transfusions of blood products given for the treatment of haemophilia. This was in the very early days before tests were available to test all blood for HIV. Nowadays all blood donations are tested for HIV and other viruses. This does not mean total certainty, as in the case of the child mentioned previously.

Prevention of HIV transmission

- Practising safe sex behaviours is of utmost importance (see Chapter 2). Health education programs have emphasised the need to wear condoms during penetrative sexual activity. Condoms provide a barrier between the body secretions of someone who is HIV positive and the body of someone who is not infected.

- Health education programs have also emphasised the need for clean syringes and needles for intravenous drug addicts. A free needle exchange program is available in most large urban areas.

  Most women are given the option of being tested for HIV as part of antenatal screening. This identifies anyone who is HIV positive so that counselling can be offered and the baby tested immediately after birth.

- Breastfeeding is not advisable for a woman who is HIV positive, so special assistance would be given psychologically as well as practically to ensure that bottle feeding is established.

HIV infection and child care

Transmission

There is no evidence of transmission of HIV infection from one child to another in child-care settings or schools. HIV is not spread through normal social contact. The risk of transmission is extremely low, even in families where young children share toys, baths, clothes, eating utensils and hug and kiss with a sibling who is HIV positive.

Many parents and staff worry about episodes of biting among toddlers, but here again the risk is minimal. The virus does not live easily in saliva and is rarely transmitted this way.

The other main concern is about cuts and grazes causing bleeding. It is recommended that staff wear gloves when attending to blood and other body discharges such as vomitus and faeces. This procedure protects both staff and children.

Confidentiality

In all situations any information given in confidence to child-care staff by parents, or anything a child tells staff, must be kept strictly confidential and not shared with anyone else. This is an important ethical principle.

There has sometimes been a lack of understanding about HIV infection and the way it is transmitted. This has meant that some staff and parents have been unwilling to accept children who are HIV positive into child-care settings. There have, in the past, been some instances where families have faced hostility and discrimination when they informed the care setting of the HIV status of their child.

Because the risk of transmission is so very low, and the risk of social discrimination so high, it is not a requirement for parents to inform the child-care setting that a child is HIV positive. The same conditions apply to staff: there is also no requirement for other staff or parents to know the HIV status of any staff member.

In a best-practice situation, both staff and parents would be well informed about HIV infection and understand that the risks of cross-infection are minimal. In such a child-care setting the policy and practice would be such that parents would feel able to share health concerns relating to HIV and their child without fear of discrimination.

Care of the child

The best possible care of the child would involve the parents, the child-care staff and the health professionals working together. Child-care staff would then be kept informed of the health profile of the child. It is best if a child is treated with anti-viral drugs as soon as he/she is found to be HIV positive.

The child will have special health needs.

- Children who are HIV positive may need to stay home if there are outbreaks of infectious diseases such as chickenpox.
- The treatment may have side effects which need to be noted.
- The child and the family will need emotional and social support.
- The child may need frequent periods of hospitalisation and need support to cope with these experiences.
- Immunisation should be given on medical advice.

Precautions to prevent cross-infection

- General preventive measures to prevent cross-infection (see Chapter 6) should be in place in all child-care settings whether there is a child who is HIV positive attending or not. These precautions will prevent the transmission of HIV and hepatitis B and C
- As a special precaution, open wounds on any child should be covered with a waterproof dressing.

Health education and HIV/AIDS

An understanding of HIV infection and AIDS is important for several reasons:

- It helps prevent the spread of HIV infection because informed people know how to take preventive measures.

- It helps toward forming a rational response to the disease rather than an emotional over-reaction.
- It encourages a better understanding of those persons who are HIV positive, which in turn helps give improved support.

Learning activities

1. List the ways that infection can be spread in a child-care setting.
2. Suggest ten specific ways to prevent cross-infection when you have a group of children together.
3. Suggest some learning experiences for toddlers and 3–5-year-olds that will encourage personal hygiene practices.
4. Find out about the availability of immunisation programs in your area.

References

Boswell JG, Nienhuys TG. (1995 Jul). Onset of otitis media in the first eight weeks of life in aboriginal and non-aboriginal Australian infants. *Ann Otol Rhino Laryngol.* 104(7):542–549.

Commonwealth Department of Health (1995). Statement on immunisation.

NHMRC (1999). *Recommended immunisation schedule (0–6 years) and (10–65+ years)*. Canberra, AGPS.

NHMRC (1997). *Staying healthy in child care.* Canberra, AGPS.

Roberts LA, Patel MS, Smith WT, Jorm LR, Douglas RM. (1999). Infection control measures reduce diarrhoeal and acute respiratory infections in child care. Paper presented at the Australian Society for Infectious Diseases conference, Cairns, April.

Skull SA, Morris PS, Yonovitz A, Attewell RG, Krause V, Leach AJ, Anand A, Scott J, Reid S, Roberts LA. (1999 Aug). Middle ear effusion: rate and risk factors in Australian children attending day care. *Epidemiol Infect* (123):57–64

Video: Department of Community Paediatrics (1998). *Calling the shots.* Royal Children's Hospital, Melbourne.

Further reading

Donowitz L, ed. (1991). *Infection control in the child care center and preschool.* Baltimore, Williams and Wilkins.

Commonwealth Department of Health and Aged Care (2000). *Understanding childhood immunisation.* Canberra, AGPS.

CHAPTER 6

Hygiene practices and health care routines

ONE OF THE important tasks in any children's service is to do all that is possible to prevent the spread of infection. Germs cannot be totally eliminated from a child-care setting, as all persons within the setting will carry some germs. The number of germs can, however, be drastically reduced which is a necessary step toward preventing infection and illness amongst children and staff. Children's services need to provide both a healthy environment and a healthy program.

Providing a healthy environment

Physical environment

The child-care setting should be arranged with health care and infection control as a priority. Ideally, all buildings used for child-care would be purpose-built and designed for the care and education of babies and young children. Toilets and bathrooms would be easily accessible to indoor and outdoor play areas, and planned in such a way that there was an uncluttered space for traffic flow and the needs of different age groups. Nappy change areas would be adjacent to babies' and toddlers' rooms and designed in such a way that they were convenient for staff and children to use, with nappy rinsing and hand-washing facilities adjacent to the change table.

Surfaces within the child-care setting would all be of materials that could easily be wiped and kept clean. Floors would have no awkward corners to collect dust and dirt. Windows could easily be opened to air rooms. Sleep rooms would be well ventilated, with adequate room to store mattresses.

Although many centres have been adapted rather than specifically designed for child care, there is much that staff can do to ensure that they are set up to enable health practices to be correctly carried out.

Grouping of children

The importance of the way that children are grouped in child-care settings (especially child-care centres) has probably been underestimated. The grouping is often done for social and educational reasons without taking the risk of infection into account.

Mixed-age groups

There is evidence that the rate of cross-infection within child-care settings is much higher when there are mixed-age groups. In particular, this happens more frequently when children who are still in nappies spend time with older children. Faecal-oral contamination can much more easily happen in this situation (NHMRC 1997).

The risk of cross-infection is highest when groups are together all day, but there are still risks when there is a mix of ages for short periods such as at the beginning and end of the day, so special care needs to be taken. This risk also applies to family day-care homes, though less so because the number of children is small.

Many people find that it is philosophically and educationally attractive to have different age groups together, but the social and other benefits of such groupings need to be carefully assessed against the possible harm caused to health.

Size of groups

There is a much higher risk of cross-infection in a child-care setting where the groups are of a large size, even if the ages are the same. Younger children, again, are at an increased risk due to their immature immune systems.

General cleaning

It is essential that there are planned procedures for general cleaning routines. These procedures are needed to limit the number of disease-causing germs on surfaces, toys and in play areas. Many child-care facilities employ a professional cleaner for the heavier tasks but child-care staff will also need to assist with cleaning procedures throughout the day.

It should be remembered that germs dislike sunlight, so that hanging articles such as mops and cleaning cloths in the sun, and opening doors and windows, help to eliminate germs from the rooms.

Cleaning solutions

A mixture of detergent and warm water is the most effective solution for general cleaning. This will wash away surface dirt that might contain disease-carrying micro-organisms. This cleaning is a very important measure for keeping children healthy.

Disinfectants will be needed for specific areas and for certain spills. Articles or surfaces must always be washed before using any disinfectant. The most effective disinfectants are quaternary ammonium compounds (quats) and diluted bleach. Labels for disinfectants should be checked carefully, as not all of them kill bacteria, viruses and fungi. Dettol and other phenol solutions kill bacteria but not viruses.

Bleach (sodium hypochlorite) is the most effective, as it kills the three types of micro-organisms, but it is essential that all surfaces be washed before diluted bleach is used. This is because direct contact with the protein in human body discharges and fluids inactivates the bleach. Solutions of diluted bleach should be made up every day; the usual strength is 1 part bleach to 9 parts water. Bleach should not be used on metal articles such as toys or cots as it has a corrosive action on metal. Gloves should be worn when using disinfectants to prevent irritation of the skin.

Cleaning routines

Floors

All floors should be swept and washed daily with detergent and warm water. Spills should be immediately wiped up during the day. Spills of blood, vomit or other body fluids should be wiped away with detergent and water and then the area cleaned with diluted bleach.

Table tops

Table tops should be wiped over daily with detergent and warm water as well as being washed after messy activities and before meal and snack times.

Other surfaces

Low shelves, doorknobs, chairs and any other surface that children frequently touch should be washed once a week.

Bathrooms

All areas of the bathroom should be cleaned daily with detergent and warm water. Special care should be taken with doorknobs, toilet flush knobs and taps, as children frequently touch these places with contaminated hands.

There should be regular checks on the bathroom during the day, eg. after hand-washing times to ensure there are no spills. Taps, toilet flush handles and doorknobs should be wiped over at these times too.

Kitchen

Any area where food is prepared should be kept scrupulously clean. It is best to have a wash basin, soap and disposable towels in the kitchen so that staff can easily wash their hands before preparing food. There is more detail about food preparation in Chapter 8.

Sleeping equipment

Children should have their own cots, stretchers, mattresses and linen and these should be washed once a week. If children use different mattresses each day, then these should be washed after use with detergent and warm water.

Linen

Linen should be washed in hot water with a laundry detergent and dried in the sun or hot clothes drier. Soiled linen should be treated in the same way as soiled nappies and soaked in diluted bleach, then washed separately in hot water. It is important for staff not to contaminate their own clothes or hands when carrying soiled linen.

Clothing

Staff clothing can become contaminated with germs, which can then infect the staff member's own family. All used clothes should be washed daily in hot water and a laundry detergent. It is a good idea to have clothes that are used solely for work, such as t-shirts in summer and windcheaters in winter. It is even better if these clothes are changed before leaving the child-care centre.

Children's clothing that is soiled should be rinsed if the soiling is bad and sent home in a securely tied plastic bag.

Dress-up clothes

These are a very important prop for dramatic play, but they can be a source of cross-infection by body contact. Dress-ups should be washed each week and if possible hung in the sun to dry. Hats should be aired in the sun.

Nappy change tables and mats

These must be washed with detergent and warm water after each use. They need to be wiped over with quaternary disinfectant or diluted bleach at the end of each morning and afternoon (or if soiled with faeces at any nappy change) and allowed to dry, if possible in the sun.

Toys

All toys used in a child-care facility should be washable. If a child has a favourite soft toy from home this should be kept in the child's cot for sleep time or used to provide comfort without being shared by other children.

Soft toys purchased by the centre should be washable. Many of these toys can go into the washing machine and be dried in the sun. Cloth books can be washed with detergent and water and also dried in the sun.

Plastic toys can be washed in the dishwasher or hand-washed in warm water and detergent.

Small toys and rattles that are being used by babies and toddlers, who still explore toys by sucking, should be washed in soap and water and then soaked in a diluted solution of Milton or other sterilising solution. There should be enough of these toys to be able to rotate them several times a day. This will not get rid of all the micro-organisms, but it will minimise the number of germs going into the babies' mouths and thus lower the rate of cross-infection.

Some child-care centres have set up a 'sin-bin' (Roberts et al. 1999) procedure where toys are placed until they are cleaned and can be returned to the babies.

Dummies (pacifiers)

These are sometimes dropped on the floor and picked up by other children, who then put them in their mouth. The whereabouts of dummies should be noted, and when not being used they should be washed, rinsed and then soaked in sterilising solution. An individual sterilising container for each child should be used.

Sandpits

Sandpits are very popular places for play, but they are a source of infection if they become contaminated by faeces and urine from cats or children. Sandpits need to be well constructed and have good drainage. They should be raked daily and covered at all times when not in use. The sand should be disinfected regularly (eg. once a month) by sprinkling with diluted bleach and raking.

Wading pools

These are often quite a joy on a hot Australian day, but they can be a serious source of infection. Wading pools must be kept clean and chlorinated in order to kill disease-causing micro-organisms.

There are many disease-causing micro-organisms in a wading pool where there are young children. Any germs from around the anal area—and there are always some there—will wash off in the wading pool and make the water very infectious. If the water is not chlorinated, then children will be very likely to get gastro-diarrhoeal diseases that can be serious. Germs from nasal discharges and open sores can also contaminate the water.

The staff can also be at risk of disease. A few years ago there were several cases of Hepatitis A among staff and parents at a child-care centre. The infectious diseases surveillance team from the local Health Department traced the source of infection back to the unchlorinated wading pool in the centre. Hepatitis A (see Chapter 5) is spread by faecal-oral means and children who are infected generally show no signs of having the disease, although they can transmit it to others. Adults who have the disease are often ill for some time.

The children

- Children who have diarrhoea, vomiting, nasal discharges or open sores should not use the wading pool.
- All children should wear clean bathers or underclothes in the pool. This will lessen the contamination.
- Get children to go to the toilet (and wash their hands) before getting into the wading pool.

- If a child defecates in the water, all the children must get out, the pool must be immediately emptied, cleaned and disinfected.

The pool

- The empty pool must be cleaned and disinfected before filling. All leaves and dust must be hosed away and the pool scrubbed out with a stiff broom and disinfectant. The disinfectant must be hosed away so there is no chance of it interacting with the chlorine.
- The pool should then be filled from the tap and the correct amount of chlorine added as it fills. The type and amount of chlorine used needs to be calculated according to the amount of water in the pool. It is important to get the right amount of chlorine for the volume of the pool: too little will not kill the germs and too much could harm the eyes and skin of the children (NHMRC 1997).

Special note

Safety is of utmost importance when using wading pools (see Chapter 8). Each State and Territory has its own regulations and some authorities may not permit the use of wading pools within a child care service.

Animals

Having animals in a child-care setting can be valuable for children. Keeping animals encourages a sense of responsibility in children as they feed and care for the pets, but some health safeguards are necessary in order to prevent infection.

- The animals should be kept healthy and veterinary advice sought if the animal is unwell in any way.
- Animals need to be kept free of parasites, so some will need de-fleaing and worming regularly. In rural areas where dogs may eat sheep offal there is a risk that hydatid tapeworm, which causes a serious disease of the liver, can be carried in the faeces of dogs.
- Cages and pens should be cleaned out regularly and faeces (apart from those in litter trays) flushed down the toilet. Litter can be placed in a paper bag and put into the rubbish tin. Particular care should be taken not to inhale the dried up faeces found on the bottom of bird cages, as this can cause psittacosis (a lung disease).

Cat faeces can cause toxoplasmosis in pregnant women and this may damage the nervous system of the fetus. Animal faeces should be kept away from sandpits and vegetable gardens.

- Animals and children should not be together while the children are eating.
- Children and caregivers must wash their hands after touching the animals.

Providing a healthy program

There is sometimes a tendency in child-care settings that health routines are seen as something separate from the other activities or learning experiences provided for the children.

The health routines within any setting should be an integral part of the learning experiences of the child. Care and education should be totally linked so that any caring routine for an infant or child is a potential learning experience.

Daily routines

The role of the caregiver when planning and implementing hygiene routines is twofold. Firstly, it is to provide essential preventive measures that will limit the spread of infection from adult to child, child to adult and child to child. Secondly, it is to provide an ongoing health education focus relating to personal hygiene and the young child. This focus should not be a separate part of the program but, rather, part of the everyday activities of the children.

Daily routines that are set in place to prevent cross-infection provide a wonderful opportunity for health education as well as enhancing other learning experiences with babies and children. The routines need to be familiar and consistent in order to provide the child with a sense of security. They should not, however, be so rigid that they ignore the changing needs of the developing child.

It is important that there is no sense conveyed that germs and dirt have negative connotations. The hygiene message should be free of value judgments, so that a child does not associate defecation or other body excretions as relating to her being 'dirty'. The excretions themselves contain germs that must be prevented from spreading, but this is not related to the worth of the child.

Children learn best from caregivers who understand the reasons for the routines and who provide good examples of infection prevention practices themselves.

Hand washing

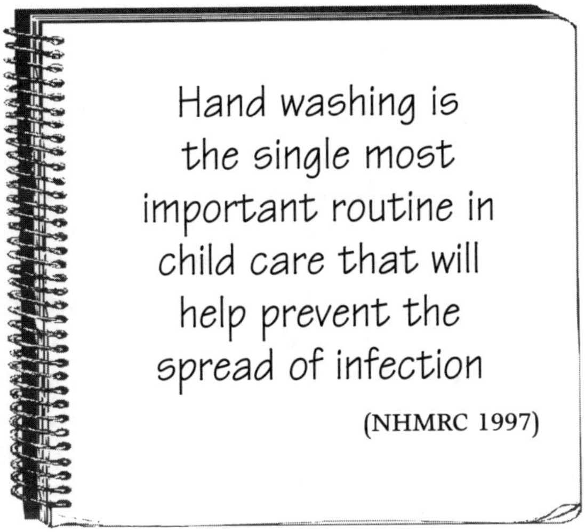
Hand washing is the single most important routine in child care that will help prevent the spread of infection
(NHMRC 1997)

This message is so important and so basic and yet it is all too often forgotten. Hand washing should always be a valuable learning experience rather than just something that needs to be done as quickly as possible before lunch and at other times in the day.

Caregivers' hands should be washed:

- On arrival at the child-care setting. This helps reduce the pool of germs that may enter the setting.
- Before any food is handled—either preparing or serving.
- Before eating.
- After changing a nappy—even when gloves have been worn.
- After going to the toilet.
- After cleaning up vomit, faeces or other body spills.
- After wiping your nose, or a child's.
- Before going home, so that germs from child care are not taken to other places and people.

Children should wash their hands:

- On arrival at child care.
- Before eating anything.
- After nappy changing, in case the child's hands have become contaminated.
- After going to the toilet.

- After playing outside.
- After playing with animals.
- After wiping nose or wiping nose secretions.
- Before going home. (NHMRC 1997)

The effectiveness of hand washing in preventing the spread of infection is dependent on the way hands are washed. It is not enough to simply run the hands under water. Hand washing is only effective when the germs on the hands are diluted and washed away together with any contaminated material that might be on the hands.

Hands should be rubbed with soap and running water for ten seconds. All surfaces including under the fingernails and between the fingers should be rubbed, as germs like to live in warm, dark, grimy places such as these. After washing, the hands should be rinsed well for ten seconds and the tap turned off with a clean paper towel, which is then discarded. The hands are then dried with a hot air drier, a disposable paper towel or an individual cloth towel that is for the use of only that child (NHMRC 1997).

Hand washing should not be a boring chore that has to be done, but a vital activity that is encouraged by songs and chants. Toddlers can sing about their fingers as they wash, and counting games used to ensure that hands are washed for long enough. There are many songs about washing hands, and caregivers and children can also make up their own. Stories with washing in them, such as *Harry the dirty dog* (Zion 1992), will allow the children to share other experiences and extend language opportunities too.

Nappy changing

Nappy changing gives the caregiver and child an opportunity for one-to-one contact. Young babies can be engaged during nappy changing by eye contact and the caregiver's voice. Wriggling older babies may need to have other distractions such as pictures or a mobile above the change table, while toddlers who are used to the routine will enjoy the attention of the caregiver. It is generally a good idea for children not to handle toys during the nappy-changing routine as the hands and toys can become contaminated with faeces or urine. Children who are still wearing nappies are often still at the developmental stage of mouthing toys, which increases the risk of contamination. Safety is also an important consideration when changing nappies, and it is essential that the caregiver always have one hand on the baby or child. Falling off change tables can cause serious injuries to the child.

There must be an area in the child-care setting that is set aside only for nappy changing. The bench or table where the changing occurs should be of a height that is comfortable for the caregivers. The table should be covered with a mat that is of a non-porous material that can be wiped down with diluted bleach solution. All equipment, lotions and clean clothes should be available within easy reach.

It is important that the correct procedure for changing nappies be carried out each time.

- Check that all articles that are needed are ready on the change table.
- Carry a baby to the change table away from your body so that your clothes do not become contaminated.
- Get a toddler to walk if possible, though a distressed child may need to be carried without contaminating your clothes.
- Place some paper on the nappy change table where the child's bottom will be placed. This paper can be recycled computer paper or any other type of suitable paper. The paper is to give extra protection, as any smeared faeces will be caught on the paper and discarded.
- Place the baby on the change table, making sure her bottom is on the paper. Older children may need to be lifted, though some children can use steps if these are provided.
- Disposable gloves must be used if the child has defecated, though many child-care settings now have policies that insist on gloves for all nappy changes. The gloves prevent any micro-organisms in the faeces from getting onto the hands or into the caregiver's body through any cracks in the skin.
- Remove all the soiled clothes and nappy and place in a plastic bag.
- Carefully clean the child's bottom with a damp paper towel and discard the towel into the bin.
- Gently lift the baby's bottom, remove the paper and place in the bin.
- Remove gloves, taking care not to touch the outside of the glove with your skin. Discard the gloves in the bin.
- Put the clean nappy on and dress the baby.
- Give the child a cuddle.
- WASH THE CHILD'S HANDS.
- Take the child away from the change table to a caregiver in another area.
- Wipe the change table over with detergent and warm water or one of the quaternary compounds.
- WASH YOUR HANDS.

Soiled nappies may need to be scraped, rinsed and soaked before being washed in the centre (or a commercial laundry) or tied up securely in a plastic bag to be sent home. Reusable rubber gloves can be kept specifically for this cleaning purpose. Some child-care settings have a slop-hopper (sluice) for rinsing nappies. Staff should wear a plastic apron while doing this so that their clothes are not contaminated. The apron should also be wiped over with detergent and water after each use, and with diluted bleach at the end of each day (NHMRC 1997).

Types of nappies

Nappies sometimes become loose when children begin to crawl and walk. This means that excreta can leak out and contaminate surfaces. Cross-infection can also occur when children in nappies sit on chairs or the floor and then another child touches this area. For this reason, many child-care settings choose to use disposable nappies while the child is in child care. Disposable nappies have a plastic covering that prevents leakage and thus reduces the risk of cross-infection.

Nappy covers should be used when cloth nappies are used. These covers ought to fit snugly and be of the wrap-round style. Elasticised pants used over nappies may, when pulled down, cause the legs and feet to become contaminated.

Toilet learning

Our culture tends to place a lot of importance on children being able to recognise, and act upon, the body feelings that signal the need to go to the toilet. It is certainly less messy for parents and caregivers to have a child who is continent and not in nappies. It also reduces the risk of cross-infection when the child is able to go to the toilet.

There is, however, enormous individual variation as to when this happens, and each child's own stage of development must be respected, as must the wishes of parents. There is no way that toilet learning can be hurried, as the main trigger to it all happening is the maturation of the nervous system. A child must make the link between certain feelings and the process and results of urination and defecation. Some children will want to feel the urine and faeces, but this should be gently discouraged by simple, calm explanations and by quickly providing alternative activities.

Most children begin toilet learning on a pot, which should be treated in exactly the same way as a fixed toilet. It should be kept in the bathroom and not brought into playrooms. It should be emptied into the toilet and not into a hand-washing bowl, though it can be washed in a trough or sluice where nappies are rinsed. Where a toilet chair is used, the chair should be wiped over after each use.

Hand washing should happen as though the child had used the toilet, and the same encouragement and explanations given. Toilet learning does not happen in a rush and the young child may need to wear appropriate protective pants for some time. Tact and sensitivity on the part of caregivers is needed during the toilet learning period, where progress is praised and reassurance given when needed. A supply of clean clothes from home can help minimise any potential fuss.

Nose wiping

The high rate of respiratory infections among young children in child care means that there are often many discharging noses. The discharge is infectious and should be gently wiped away with a clean disposable tissue in order to prevent the infection spreading. Dried up discharges from unwiped noses can also spread infection to other children. An older child can wipe his nose himself, while younger children will need an explanation of what is happening before a caregiver wipes the nose. Soiled tissues are put into a covered bin. Hands must be washed immediately after nose wiping.

Noses often need to be wiped when children are in areas such as the sandpit or other outdoor areas where there are no hand-washing facilities.

The best method of wiping noses in situations where hand-washing is impossible is to use cheap small plastic sandwich bags. These are much cheaper than using disposable gloves, which might be an alternative solution. The tissue is put into the bag and the nose wiped, with the caregiver only touching the outside of the bag. The tissue and bag are then disposed of into a covered container (Roberts et al. 1999).

Sunscreen application

This is also a routine that can spread infection. Children often go outside in groups and the sunscreen lotion is put onto faces and bodies, one child after the other. It would be very difficult to wash hands in between each child, but there is a real risk of infection from micro-organisms around the nose and mouth being spread from one child to another. It is possible that nasal discharges are spread from one child to another in this way. Using a separate cotton ball as a sunscreen applicator for each child would prevent contamination and spread of infection.

Another suggestion is to have small pieces of soft cloth that can be used for a single child then put into a stocking bag and washed for reuse (Roberts et al. 1999).

Teeth cleaning

This is an important health routine and one that needs to be established in early childhood. Special care needs to be taken within group care situations to ensure that cross-infection does not occur.

The membrane covering the gums is very fragile and easily broken when cleaning teeth. This means that toothbrushes can become contaminated with blood as well as saliva. It is conceivable that diseases such as Hepatitis B and C could be transmitted by toothbrushes coming into contact with one another.

For this reason, it is essential for each child to have his/her own toothbrush and that each toothbrush is rinsed and stored quite separately. It is very unsafe to put all toothbrushes together in a bowl of sterilising solution, as it is impossible to ensure that all the surfaces of all the bristles will be in contact with the solution. Toothbrushes are often stored or hung up very close together, which means that it is possible, even after they have been rinsed, for infected drips from some brushes to contaminate others.

Some child-care settings have decided to omit teeth cleaning at lunchtime. This is because they consider that the risk of cross-infection is greater than any disadvantage created by a gap in training in dental hygiene. This is a decision that needs to be discussed with parents and local dentists. If teeth cleaning is not carried out, then children should rinse their mouth to remove any debris left after eating.

Health education

Babies

Babies are dependent on adults for all personal hygiene routines such as bathing, clean clothes and nappy changing. Hygiene routines form an important part of the planned learning experiences. Babies learn in many ways, not least by relating certain activities to pleasant experiences. The baby who has a happy bathtime, where he can kick and splash and where a caregiver responds by talking, singing and smiling, will start relating this hygiene routine with positive feelings. Bathtime is not just a routine where the grime of the day is removed, but a time for sharing and closeness.

It is important to assess all hygiene routines to see if they can offer the opportunity to enhance and extend other areas of development. Asking the question, 'How can this routine be a valuable learning experience for the child?' often suggests new approaches to hygiene routines.

Nappy changing can be used as an example. It is primarily a routine to remove the soilings of excreta for health and comfort, but it offers possibilities for so much more. The experiences provided for the baby during nappy changing should promote every area of development.

Physical development

Nappy changing promotes physical development by ensuring a healthy environment that prevents cross-infection. It also helps keep the child comfortable and clean. A child who is uncomfortable will be miserable, and a child who is not clean is at risk of infections that may well affect growth. Nappy changing also allows babies to kick their legs freely without the constraints of nappies and this assists with gross motor development.

Intellectual development

Talking with the baby while changing the nappy encourages language development and communication. Caregivers also describe to children what they are doing during the changing, which extends understanding and cognitive development.

Social development

Nappy changing provides an ideal opportunity for social interaction. The caregiver is necessarily physically close to the child and there will be smiles and eye contact, together with verbal interaction. Verbal interaction includes the noises that babies make before they can speak.

Emotional development

Nappy changing is a time for one-to-one attention, with lots of eye contact and a cuddle at the end of the routine.

Washing babies' hands

Washing the baby's hands after nappy changing is obviously necessary if the baby has contaminated his hands. Washing hands as part of the routine after every nappy change reinforces the pattern of behaviour that is needed for personal hygiene. A young baby's hands can be wiped with an individual soft wet cloth, an older baby can be tucked under the caregiver's arm and have his hands washed under the tap in a basin. The caregiver should chat about what is happening while wiping or washing the baby's hands.

Toddlers (12 months to $2\frac{1}{2}$ years of age)

It is necessary to sensitively balance the toddler's increasing need for independence and her cognitive and physical ability to carry out tasks. An older toddler may be able to go to the toilet with minimal assistance but not have the necessary manipulative skills to adequately clean herself of smeared faeces around the anal area. A toddler will almost certainly want to press the flush button herself and turn the tap on for washing hands.

This independence is a very important part of a child's development and should be encouraged. Yet the need to prevent the spread of infection is equally important. The case study on page 124 in Chapter 5 showed how easy it is for faecal-oral contamination to occur with toddlers in a child-care setting.

Recognising the toddler's stage of development means that caregivers can encourage independence while promoting positive hygiene pratices. A sensitive caregiver will not intrude but offer assistance when required, while gently explaining why bottoms need wiping and hands need washing. The caregiver will understand the need for supervision in the bathroom to ensure that hygiene procedures are properly carried out.

Toddlers can also extend their experiences relating to personal hygiene by activities such as washing of dolls, clothes and home corner dishes. Many other developmental areas are enhanced, such as social interaction and co-operation, fine and gross motor skills, together with opportunities for language and cognitive enhancement. 'Real' tasks such as wiping the tables are also important, as this promotes a proper sense of self-esteem.

Stories can also be used to promote not only language and cognitive development but also personal hygiene. Sharing the familiar domestic experiences of the child in books such as Ormerod's *Sunshine* and *Moonlight* gives lots of opportunities for the toddler and caregiver to discuss many hygiene routines in an interesting and direct way (see 'Books for Reading with Children' at the end of this chapter).

Caregivers also need to be alert to any possibilities where hygiene messages can be reinforced. Although toddlers are generally not able to cognitively grasp the concept of germs and their spread, they are able to recognise and anticipate regular routines.

Three-to-five-year-olds

Children in this age group are beginning to develop the cognitive skills needed to understand the idea of germs and their spread. They can see droplets form if they breathe on a mirror and understand that the droplets contain germs that spread when they cough and sneeze over others. They can understand that the thistledown or dandelion puffball that flies off into the wind when they blow it is rather like the way that germs spread. They know that there are very small and very big things and that some things are so small you need a magnifying glass to see them. Science activities will have included looking through magnifying glasses.

Hygiene routines are now also very well established and the child understands why they are important. The child's increasing manipulative skills also mean that she can carry out nose wiping, bottom wiping and other routines herself. She will need occasional gentle reminders, because there will be times when she rushes in for lunch after an exciting activity outside and be so hungry that she forgets to count to ten as she washes her hands. The program of the child-care setting will take the exuberant 3-to-5-year-old into account and plan a quieter transitional period that spans the time from energetic activities to mealtimes, and it is in this quieter time that hand washing happens.

There will also be lots of songs, chants and stories that relate to hygiene. Some of these songs and chants will come from the children and include made-up words. Dramatic play opportunities on a health theme can reinforce hygiene messages. Visitors from a range of health professions such as community-health nursing can talk with the children about infection and other health topics. Posters and pictures depicting positive hygiene practices can be displayed.

Six-to-twelve-year-olds

It is still important to reinforce personal hygiene practices, even though children within this age range now have real knowledge of how diseases are spread. It is important that out-of-school care should continue to promote hygiene practices. Hand washing is still important and soap will need to be supplied.

Children in the older age range of this group are forming very close friendships and often want to find rituals to celebrate this friendship. In the past some children have chosen to become 'blood' brothers or sisters by cutting their skin and mixing the blood. This is now a potential method for transmission of diseases that are spread through blood, and so must be positively discouraged, as should giving each other tattoos.

Health care of infants and the growing child

The health routines that help to prevent cross-infection have been discussed in the first part of this chapter, but there are many other care routines that help keep the child healthy and which offer opportunities for positive learning experiences.

Babies

Bathing

This can be a delightful routine for both caregivers and children. Infants and younger babies are best bathed in a baby bath on a stand or table that is a comfortable height for the caregiver. Older babies and toddlers enjoy splashing with toys in a full-size bath, though this means that the caregiver needs to kneel down to be near the child. Some child-care settings have hand-held showers in a specially fitted bath and these are useful for washing an older baby or toddler who is covered with sand or dirt or is very messy with faeces, as it means the child does not have to sit in the contaminating substance. Some young children find a shower distressing, and these preferences need to be taken into account.

Routine bathing is usually done daily, though the time of day is dependent on the baby's needs and the family or child-care routine. Some parents will choose to bath a baby in the evening so that both parents can share the enjoyment. Toddlers and older children usually need to be bathed in the evening to get rid of the accumulated grime of the day.

Caregivers need to prepare the bath and ensure that all articles likely to be required are ready before the baby or child is brought to the bath. This includes testing the temperature of the water. A general rule is that the cold water should be put into the bath first, as this prevents heat being absorbed into the surface of the bath and thus burning the baby's tender skin. In many care settings a thermometer would be used to check the temperature, though more often the caregiver will check that the water is not too hot or cold by placing her elbow (where the skin is sensitive) in the water. The water should feel warm but not hot.

Bathing young babies

The articles needed for bathing a baby will include:

- Soap or baby wash lotion to put into bath water.
- Soft face flannel and towel.
- Cotton balls for wiping face.
- Any lotions such as baby oil for massage or cream to prevent nappy rash.
- Clean clothes and nappy.
- Container for dirty clothes and soiled nappies.
- Soft brush for hair.

Hannah is working in a private home, where she is responsible for the care of Jessy who is 3 months old. Jessy's parents are both employed full-time, though her mother comes home each day at lunchtime to give her a breast feed. Sometimes she can get home in time to bath Jessy, though usually Hannah does this.

Jessy usually sleeps from mid- to late morning and has her bath when she wakes. She is usually happy to wait for her feed at this time. Hannah checks that the room is a comfortable temperature and gets the bath items ready before Jessy wakes and has all she needs, apart from the water in the bath. Hannah is very alert to the first stirrings of Jessy and allows her to fully wake up before she puts water and cleansing lotion in the bath and checks the temperature. She then greets Jessy and picks her up from the cot, chatting gently as she does so.

Jessy enjoys her bath, though she doesn't like being undressed. Hannah is adept at taking off the baby's clothes without covering Jessy's face and she smiles and sings to Jessy as she does so. Jessy gurgles and smiles in return. All the clothes are removed (and placed in a soiled-linen bucket) apart from the nappy, so that Jessy's face and hair can be washed without fear of contamination. Hannah uses single cotton balls to gently wipe Jessy's eyes from the inner to outer edge and makes sure she gets into all the crevices behind Jessy's ears and in the ear lobe. This is an area where sores can form if not cleaned and dried properly.

Hannah wraps Jessy in a towel and tucks the baby under her arm in order to wash Jessy's hair. She uses a very mild baby shampoo and has a small plastic jug of warm water from the bath to rinse the hair. Much care is taken not to get either the shampoo or rinsing water near Jessy's eyes. The hair is also patted with the towel to prevent it dripping when Jessy is in the bath.

The nappy is removed next and dropped into a nappy bucket. The nappy clasp is placed where Jessy cannot reach it and scratch herself. The room is warm and comfortable and Jessy kicks and kicks and it is sometimes difficult to pick her up and get her into the bath. Hanna laughs with Jessy as she lifts her into the water, laying the baby in the crook of her arm and leaving Jessy's legs and arms free to splash in the water. There is no hurry as long as the water stays warm, and Hannah washes Jessy slowly with a soft face flannel, observing Jessy's skin and chatting with her as she does so. Hannah and Jessy both enjoy this time together. Sometimes Hannah sings songs and chants rhymes such as Head and shoulders, knees and toes *(*Merrily merrily songbook*).*

Continued

Hannah lifts Jessy out of the bath onto the towel and softly dries the baby, making sure that all the skin folds are completely dry, as dampness can chafe the skin and allow germs to enter. There is a little redness in Jessy's groin area so Hannah very carefully dries this part and then softly rubs some zinc cream into the skin. Toenails and fingernails are also checked at this time.

Jessy's parents do not use talc powder but have shown Hannah how to massage the baby with some baby oil, which is very lightly scented. Jessy almost flops in relaxation as Hannah gently massages the oil into her body. Jessy is quite dreamy about being dressed, though Hannah again ensures that her face is not covered while her clothes are put on and her hair brushed.

Clean, dry and dressed, Jessy is safely tucked into her bouncinette in a safe place on the floor while Hannah cleans up the bathing equipment and changes the bedclothes on the cot. Soon Jessy's mother will be home to feed her. Hannah will cuddle and chat with Jessy until that time.

Toddlers and older babies who are sitting well without support enjoy having containers that can be filled and emptied and which will float and sink. These activities make bathtime a valuable science experience as well as a necessary hygiene routine.

Caregivers must always STAY WITH the baby or young child during bathtime. There is always the risk of drowning, even in very small amounts of water, and older babies and young children can slip over and hit their head.

Skin care

Babies are often prone to non-specific rashes, as their skin is sensitive. Very young babies may develop tiny pustules on their face, which clear up of their own accord. Heat rash can be a bother for babies in hot, humid climates; this problem can be reduced by keeping the child in light cotton clothes and drying the baby as well as possible between all skin folds and creases such as the toes, under arms and around the neck. Special zinc oxide powder formulated for babies can sometimes soothe the rash, together with tepid washes and changing the clothes several times a day.

Nappy rash is caused by ammonia from wet nappies and from a reaction to soap powder or other washing solution which has not been adequately rinsed from the nappies. It is recommended that nappies be soaked in one of the sodium hypochlorite solutions specifically made for that purpose before being washed in very mild soap and thoroughly rinsed. Babies should not be left in wet nappies; frequent changes are essential. Plastic pants may trap the ammoniac moisture near a baby's skin and thus cause nappy rash.

Sunlight acting on molecules in the skin is a source of Vitamin D, but the harsh sun of Australia can cause serious burns to the skin of children. Being sunburnt in childhood increases the risk of skin cancers and melanoma in adult life. All children, and caregivers too, should wear protective clothing such as a hat and t-shirt as well as using a 15+ sunscreen. The program of the child-care setting should reinforce that this is an important routine before going out into the sun. Role modelling on the part of staff is one way of reinforcing this learning. It is a good idea to plan activities in the shade during the hottest hours of a summer day.

Hair care

Young babies do not need to have their hair washed every day, though many parents will choose to do this. A very mild baby shampoo that does not sting the eyes can be used. A mild conditioner may prevent tangles as the hair grows thicker and longer.

Sometimes the skin secretes too much sebum onto the scalp and a dried up browny-yellow crust, commonly known as cradle cap, appears on the scalp. This is a type of dermatitis. One treatment is to soften the crust with baby oil so that it can be washed off. There are many other available lotions that can be used.

Clothes

Clothes are an important part of culture and personal values, as well as serving to keep people warm in winter and cool in summer. Children need clothes in which they can be active and which are comfortable and safe.

The wishes of parents regarding dress should be respected while still making sure that there is adequate communication with parents about the activities programmed for each group of children. Open discussion with parents about the value to the child and the learning that happens during sand play, climbing and messy activities encourages parents to be involved and choose appropriate clothes for their children.

Most child-care settings request that spare clothes for each child be brought to child care each day. All clothes should be clearly labelled with the child's name. Children's clothes are expensive and staff can show respect for the parents and care for the child by ensuring as far as possible that clothes are not lost and are put into the correct bags to be sent home for washing. Smocks and other protective clothing should be supplied for messy activities, and the paints and dyes used should all be washable.

Parental values and reasons for dress may not be always be obvious to child-care staff, as in the case of a professional Aboriginal woman who insisted that her child be spotlessly clean both in clothes and person before leaving the child-care centre. The director of the centre had a good relationship with this parent and one day asked why the child needed to be so very clean. The mother then explained that she caught public transport and one day when her child had on a paint-stained dress, she was dismayed and humiliated to overhear another passenger say, 'Look at that Aboriginal woman and her dirty child'.

The Aboriginal woman felt that the only way she could tackle such overt racism was to ensure that her child always be so clean that such criticism could not happen again. An empathetic child-care staff helped her with this by having her child neat and clean at the end of each day.

Babies

Babies' clothes are best made from natural fibres that can easily be soaked and washed. They need to be of a design that makes for ease when changing nappies, and have head holes large enough to get over a baby's head without having to tug or cover the baby's face. Baby clothes are also best without ribbons and other decorative tassels that can be swallowed or get caught and cause choking or strangulation.

All-in-one jump suits are very practical for young babies as they have built-in feet and thus there is no need for socks or booties, which tend to be kicked off. It is important to make sure that there is plenty of room in the suits to allow for both movement and growth.

Crawlers

Once a baby has begun to crawl she will get into all sorts of places and her clothes will get dirty. Clothes need to be made of fabric strong enough to withstand heavy washing. Again, as with younger babies, the design needs to allow for easy nappy changing and the necks of jumpers and t-shirts should be large enough, or have clip fastenings, so that a child is not distressed getting her head into and out of such garments. Crawlers also need clothes that do not hinder their movement: girls frequently get caught up in dresses, so trousers are best for both genders, though it is important to acknowledge cultural influences on dress.

The style of clothes will also be dependent on the type of floor coverings upon which a child crawls. A scratchy surface such as matting will require long trousers, while bare knees may be fine on soft carpet. Shoes are generally not needed until the child is walking outside, but warm socks may be needed in cold weather.

Toddlers

Children of this age will start to have preferences for specific clothes and may want to wear the same t-shirt day after day. Caregivers may find that none of the t-shirts in the child's bag is acceptable if the favourite shirt becomes wet or very dirty.

The need to explore means that toddlers will be best in clothes that allow for lots of movement. Long dresses can cause girls to trip when they stand up, and dresses can get caught in climbing equipment and cause falls. Again, there needs to be respect for cultural differences and for parental values concerning dress. A compromise can sometimes be reached where children change into practical clothing when they come to the child-care setting and change again before going home. This should only happen after discussion with parents.

A toddler's growing independence means that the child will want to dress himself, so it is important that the design of clothes helps rather than hinders this. Small buttons are difficult to manipulate, as are stiff zips. Track suits in winter and elasticised shorts and t-shirts in summer are often very practical. Velcro is useful on shoes and jackets as it is easy to manage and thus encourages self-help skills. Shoes need to be both flexible and sturdy, with non-slip soles for running and climbing.

This is also the age for toilet learning and trousers often need to be taken off. A sensitive caregiver will offer assistance when necessary but not intrude where a child is managing, albeit slowly. Giving toddlers enough time to dress is essential in order to promote self-esteem and a sense of independence at this stage of development.

Older children

Dress for older children also needs to be practical and allow for physical movement. Older children are starting to develop expression of their personality through dress, and peer group pressure and advertisements may well influence their choices. This can often be an expensive time for parents.

Sleeping patterns

All humans need times of rest and sleep though, as in most areas of human behaviour, there is a lot of individual variation as to how much is needed. Some of these variations could be related to personality traits: an outgoing boisterous child may seem to need less sleep than a quieter child.

Sleep is divided into two types:

1. Rapid eye movement (REM) which is active sleep, from which people easily awaken.
2. Non-rapid eye movement (NREM) which is deep (or quiet) sleep, from which it is much harder to be aroused.

Although there are such huge individual differences in how much sleep is needed, there are many external factors that affect the ability to sleep. Most people find it difficult to sleep in bright, noisy places and infants and children are no different. The environment should be arranged to induce rather than hinder the ability to sleep.

Infants

Most parents of young babies would say that their own sleep patterns are what change with the birth of a baby, who has yet to establish his own sleep patterns and who needs night feedings for some weeks, if not months. Some very young babies sleep soundly, waking only to feed. Others have periods of restlessness, often with crying, or they lie awake looking around at their world.

Parents and staff will discuss a baby's sleep patterns on enrolment. Family values and cultural factors, again, are important and play a big part in where babies sleep. Some families will choose to have the baby in their bed or in a pram or bassinet nearby. Babies in other families may sleep in a separate room. The actual sleeping equipment can also differ, with hammocks being used as well as bassinets, cots and prams. The design and manufacture of sleeping equipment is an important safety issue in the care of babies and young children.

The child-care environment should, as far as possible, be similar to that which the baby has at home. The baby should have her own sleeping place, with familiar and comforting toys, mobiles and other play things nearby. Familiar routines should be followed such as rocking, stroking and singing soft lullabies. Babies, as discussed in Chapter 3, should not sleep on their fronts as this increases the risk of Sudden Infant Death Syndrome (cot death). The temperature of the nursery should be neither too warm nor too cold.

The sleeping routine of each baby should be noted and discussed with parents so that individual and family needs can be met. A baby's sleep pattern will change a lot as she grows, and staff need to be observant and sensitive to these changes as they occur.

Toddlers

Once children reach about 18 months they have usually settled into a routine where a sleep after lunch is all that is needed. Some children may be more tired than others by late morning and they should be given the opportunity to be the first to have lunch and then go straight to sleep. It is a good idea to set up the staff routine so that beds are ready well before the children's nap time, and that favourite soft toys and books are placed on each child's bed. The sleep room should be quiet, well aired yet without bright light.

Regular routines are an important part of helping a toddler feel secure. The child should know what to expect when lunch is finished, and the transition period should be peaceful and positive. The familiar patterns of toiletting, hand-washing, getting undressed, knowing where to put their clothes, and where their bed is, reassures children that all is well with their world and support their sense of trust.

Some children fall asleep very quickly, others may look at picture books or cuddle a favourite soft toy. Some staff will stroke a restless child's back in order to promote relaxation and sleep.

Older children

Some children stop needing a daytime sleep by the time they are 3–4 years of age. A flexible routine within child care should enable these children to have quiet activities during the sleep time.

It can be quite difficult getting the balance right with sleep and the 3–5 year olds. Some parents find that their child does not go easily to bed at night if he has a sleep in the daytime. Child-care professionals sometimes find that the child who has not slept in the daytime is so tired by the end of the afternoon that no positive interaction or play is possible. These dilemmas need understanding discussions between parents and staff, so that the best solution for the child, family and child-care service can be found.

Other concerns

Security items

Most people have favourite possessions such as a picture, book or ornament. Many of these objects are related to particular events and bring back special memories and feelings. Children often attach very special significance to certain objects that promote a sense of security, and this is part of emotional health. Using these items seems to help to reduce anxiety during periods of mild stress.

The objects to which children become attached are very varied but are usually sensory and related to sucking and/or feelings of touch. Children start learning about their world through sensory (feeling) exploration in the time before they are able to use the abstractions of language.

A child's attachment to a dummy, soft toy, blanket or even what seems like pieces of rag is important and should be respected. Some parents and caregivers become concerned about the attachment, but should be reassured that in most cases this gets less as the child gets older.

Separation anxiety

Children naturally become very attached to their parents (or primary caregiver) and sometimes become very distressed when separated. This distress does not usually occur in the very early months, and the start may be linked to the developmental stage when children realise that objects (and people) exist even when out of sight. The advent of 'stranger shyness' at about 7–8 months makes meeting new people even more distressing.

In most situations parents are able to settle the children slowly into the care setting. The first day the parent may come for only an hour, or even less, and be with the child the whole time. The time is gradually extended until the child is familiar with the other children, staff and centre routine.

The parent might then leave the child for an hour or so, having first explained what is happening and when he will return. Young children do not have well developed concepts of time and the actual hours on the clock do not mean very much. It is clearer for the child if the parent's time of return is linked to an activity at child care such as lunchtime, after sleep or afternoon snack. The child then slowly spends more and more time in the child-care setting until fully settled.

This slow settling-in period cannot happen in an emergency where a parent has been suddenly admitted to hospital or through any other family disruption. The child in this situation has suffered the trauma of the family being disrupted, which is made worse by being in a totally strange place with unknown people. This child will need much reassurance.

Sometimes children who have been attending a child-care setting for some time suddenly start to become distressed when the parent leaves. There may be various reasons for this. Staff or routine changes can be upsetting until the child becomes used to these. Children also change as they develop, and it may be that a child needs extra reassurance while she readjusts to the child-care setting. Sometimes parents are able to stay a little longer in the mornings until the child is settled.

It is important that staff are honest with parents about how long it is taking the child to settle. The child's wellbeing is of paramount importance and this cannot be attained without trust between caregiver and parent.

Specific behavioural concerns

Biting

This happens most with toddlers who have not yet reached a stage where they are able to say how they feel, and so they demonstrate their feelings of frustration by biting. These feelings of frustration often occur when another child takes away a toy, or when they themselves want something and, lacking the language/cognitive ability to ask for it, they bite and snatch.

The emphasis should be on prevention, on trying to limit the number of frustrating situations the child experiences. This can be done by setting up the environment so that the child has access to the toys and other articles she needs and that there are enough of these toys and articles for all the children.

Biting is not acceptable behaviour and this should be gently pointed out to the child. Simple factual comments such as 'It hurts when you bite' are much more useful than placing an abstract moral emphasis on the action and saying 'That is a naughty thing to do'.

Attention should always be given to the child who has been bitten, but staff should ensure that the child who is prone to bite in a frustrating situation has plenty of attention during the day. It would be of great concern if the child only received one-to-one attention when she bit another child.

Swearing

There are some words in all languages that are considered offensive. In earlier times these words were often religious in origin and were thought to offend against God and the Church. Today's swear words are more likely to have an offensive sexual connotation.

Children learn from the behaviours and actions of others. It would be very hard for children to escape hearing words that are regarded as swearing when they are heard in the street, on the radio and television. Some parents will swear at times of exasperation and frustration, others may do so frequently.

Children start experimenting with language almost as soon as they start speaking. Around 4 years of age there may be a surge of language activity which plays with words relating to excretory bodily functions and body parts. Swearing often becomes an issue at about the same time.

Adults often react quite vehemently to children swearing. It must be very interesting to the child that using one or two words creates such a reaction. It is important, though, that children have an opportunity to learn that some actions or words are not appropriate, as this is part of socialisation.

By the time a child starts swearing, he is usually old enough to understand that there are acceptable and non-acceptable behaviours within the child-care setting. Hitting other children is considered unacceptable, as it physically hurts. In the same way, swearing is unacceptable because it hurts the feelings of other people. Setting limits in this way, and gently yet firmly reinforcing what is acceptable, is usually enough to stop the swearing occurring. The child needs to have challenging activities to do, and at which he can succeed. Parents also need to be informed of the child-care policy relating to swearing.

Learning activities

Think about settling a group of 2–3-year-olds to a rest period after lunch.

1. How would you plan for each individual child to prepare for rest? You might think of practical activities such as:
   - going to the toilet
   - nappy changing
   - hand-washing and drying
   - undressing.
2. What 'activities' might help the children settle?

3. Think about getting-up time. Can the children sleep undisturbed until they wake naturally?
4. How will you encourage independence with dressing?
5. Explore some songs and stories that could be used to enhance health routines.

References

Improving infection control in child care: infection control kit (2000). Melbourne Centre for Community Child Health, Royal Children's Hospital.

This kit is based on the work of Dr Leslee Roberts whose work we have referred to many times in Chapters 5 and 6.

The kit contains:

- a self-paced learning booklet on best practices for infection control
- a handwashing poster
- a video cassette on how to implement best infection control practices
- the video cassette *Calling the shots* on immunisation in child care.

NHMRC (1997). *Staying healthy in child-care*. Canberra, AGPS.

Nursing Mothers' Association of Australia (1983). *Merrily merrily songbook*. Melbourne, NMAA.

Roberts LA, Patel MS, Smith WT, Jorm LR, Douglas RM. Infection control measures reduce diarrhoeal and acute respiratory infections in child-care. Paper presented at the Australian Society for Infectious Diseases conference, Cairns, April 1999.

Zion G. (1992). *Harry the dirty dog*. London, Random House.

Books for reading with children

Fox M. (1993). *Time for bed*. Adelaide, Omnibus Books.

James A. (1989). *One day*. Melbourne, Oxford University Press.

Ormerod J. (1982). *Sunshine*. Melbourne, Puffin.

Ormerod J. (1983). *Moonlight*. Melbourne, Puffin.

Further reading

Bell C. (1999). *Highlighting health*. Canberra, Australian Early Childhood Association.

Donowitz LG, ed. (1991). *Infection control in the child-care center and preschool*. Baltimore, Williams and Wilkins.

Greenman J and Stonehouse A. (1997). *Prime times: A handbook for excellence in infant and toddler programs*. Sydney, Addison Wesley Longman.

Hutchins T. (1995). *Babies need more than minding*. Canberra, Australian Early Childhood Association.

NHMRC (1999). *Recommended immunisation schedule (0–6 years) and (10–65+ years)*. Canberra, AGPS.

NHMRC (1997). *Staying healthy in child-care*. Canberra, AGPS.

CHAPTER 7

Nutrition

NUTRITION IS A very serious health issue within any community. Not only do young children need enough of the right sort of foods to help them to stay healthy, be active and grow to their full potential, they also need to eat the types of foods when young that will establish a healthy pattern for adult life.

There is much evidence now that many diseases in adult life are caused by poor food choices in childhood. There is also increasing concern that the diets of many Australian children are not nutritionally sound, but are far too high in fat, salt and sugar, too low in fibre and too high in energy (NHMRC 1989). Heart disease is linked to a high intake of animal fat and salt, adult diabetes to foods that are high in sugar, and bowel cancer to a lack of fibre in the diet. High-energy foods contain too many kilojoules (or calories) and can lead to children becoming overweight, which can create a problem that can persist throughout adult life.

Food preferences and attitudes toward food begin early in life and it is therefore important that children's services not only provide a well balanced diet for all children, but that positive attitudes toward nutritious food are encouraged. Children may well be in child care for 8 hours a day, and two-thirds of their daily food requirements will need to be given in this setting. Working in partnership with parents is an essential part of a successful nutrition program for children.

Dietary guidelines for children and adolescents

These guidelines have been developed by nutritionists in order to provide Australian parents and health-care professionals with accurate information about food and health.

- Encourage and support breast-feeding.
- Children need appropriate food and physical activity to grow and develop normally. Growth should be checked regularly.
- Enjoy a wide variety of nutritious foods.
- Eat plenty of breads and cereals, vegetables (including legumes) and fruits.
- Low-fat diets are not suitable for young children. For older children, a diet low in fat and, in particular, low in saturated fat is appropriate.
- Encourage water as a drink. Alcohol is not recommended for children.
- Eat only a moderate amount of sugars and foods containing added sugars.
- Choose low salt foods.

Guidelines on specific nutrients

- Eat foods containing calcium.
- Eat foods containing iron.

NHMRC 1995

General nutrition information

Diet

The term diet simply means the food we eat. Some people may be on a special diet for weight loss or food allergy. Diets are used to control a disease, as in the case of diabetes, or to prevent a disease from developing, as in the case of phenylketonuria. Most people do not need a special diet, but rather a diet that is well balanced and which provides all the nutrients needed for the person's stage of life and level of activity. In many cultures the type of food will be different, though the necessary nutrients remain the same: rice, noodles, pasta or potato may well be consumed daily in different parts of the world. Family and religious values also play a part in the types of food eaten, and many people eat ritual or traditional foods on special occasions. Diet also changes according to season and the availability of foods.

Nutrients

Food contains nutrients (protein, carbohydrate, fat, minerals, vitamins) and water, which are needed by the body and have specific roles in maintaining health and body function, promoting growth in children and in providing energy. The same nutrients are found in a variety of foods. For example, rice, noodles, pasta or potato all contain high amounts of carbohydrate in the form of starch; fruit and vegetables contain vitamins and minerals; milk, eggs, beans and meat contain protein. So a diet that contains all the essential nutrients can come from a variety of foods. Table 7.1 explains the functions of different nutrients and describes the foods that contain them.

Energy

Children do need to have foods that provide the energy needed for activity, but these foods must also contain nutrients. The amount of energy contained in foods is measured by kilojoules (or calories). Some foods contain a lot of energy but few nutrients. These foods, such as lollies (sweets), soft drink and chips (crisps), tend to be very high in sugar or fat, which will supply energy but few nutrients. Many other foods, such as cereals and fruit, contain lots of energy, but they also contain many nutrients and satisfy hunger, unlike the empty kilojoules of lollies and crisps.

Overweight, or obesity, happens when the energy intake exceeds that which the child (or adult) puts out in the form of activity and exercise. Eating fruit, vegetables and cereals satisfies hunger without the risk of overweight; this is not the case with crisps or lollies.

What makes up a healthy diet?

There are several ways of planning a healthy diet for a child . . . and for adults too.

The five basic food groups

Another way that we can look at analysing food is to use the five basic food groups.

Table 7.2 sets out the five food groups, the nutrients each group contains and the daily amount of the food needed by children.

Table 7.1. Nutrients

Nutrient	Function	Found in	Too much	Too little
PROTEIN (animal and vegetable)	Builds new tissue and repairs old or damaged tissue Especially needed by pregnant women, babies and young children	All animal (meat, chicken, fish) and dairy foods (cheese, eggs, milk) Some vegetables especially legumes (beans, peas, nuts) Note: For children under 5 years old, nuts need to be crushed or in paste	Hard to have too much when very young. Excess protein is stored as fat in body so too much causes children to become overweight	Undernourished with poor growth, more susceptible to infections Severe protein deficiency leads to a disease called kwashiorkor which can cause death
FATS (animal and vegetable)	Provide heat and energy for body. Protect organs such as kidneys. Help insulate body Also needed to help the body use non-soluble vitamins	Saturated fats in all animal foods though most fish has less fat than beef or lamb Vegetables such as nuts and avocadoes Most vegetable oils are unsaturated fats coconut oil and palm oil are exceptions)	Small amounts contain high kilojoules so too much dietary fat causes children to become overweight	Infants and young children need an adequate amount of fat in their diet. They do not need fried or fatty foods but should be given full strength milk and other dairy products after 12 months of age until they are eating a variety of other foods containing protein and calcium Human breast milk is very high in fat which is right for babies

CARBOHYDRATES (starches and sugars)	Provide heat and energy Fibre from skins and seeds provide bulk for faeces	Starches are found in all cereals (pasta, rice, noodles, bread) and root vegetables (potatoes, carrots, swedes, turnips) Most other vegetables also contain starch Sugars are found in milk (lactose), all fruits and some vegetables (fructose) Sucrose is found in honey and sugar. Products containing sugar such as sweets and soft drink contain empty calories with no nutritional value	Excess carbohydrates are stored in the body as adipose tissue which causes obesity	Children will be underweight and their growth retarded

Continued

Table 7.1. (*Continued*)

Nutrient	Function	Found in	Too much	Too little
VITAMINS Water soluble—Vitamin B (many types) and C	Regulate specific body functions	Vitamin B—meat, poultry, fish, eggs, whole grain cereals, fruit and vegetables (especially green leafy vegetables), yeast extracts such as Vegemite Vitamin C—all fresh fruits and vegetables and especially citrus fruits and berries	Excess water-soluble vitamins are not stored in body but excreted in urine Excessive amounts of B6 can cause damage to nervous system	Too little of the Vitamin B group leads to skin rashes, wasting of muscles and heart disease. Too little folic acid in pregnancy increases the risk of spina bifida in the baby Too little Vitamin C leads to scurvy, where serious bleeding of the gums and tissues occurs
Fat soluble—Vitamins A, D, E, K	Vitamin A—healthy tissues which line eyes, ears and other body organs Vitamin D needs sunlight acting on molecules in the skin to help with bone formation	Vitamin A is found in all orange-yellow food such as carrots, pumpkin, apricot, tropical fruits. Some green leafy vegetables such as broccoli, spinach, cabbage and parsley. Vitamin A is also found in animal	Excess fat soluble vitamins are stored in the liver and can cause toxicity. It is difficult to overdose if vitamin D is gained purely by eating food but care should be taken if vitamin supplements are taken	Too little leads to unhealthy tissues, bones and a reduced ability to clot blood

	and growth Vitamin E protects cells from damage Vitamin K assists the blood to clot	foods liver, eggs, butter and cheese Vitamin D provided by sunlight and fish liver oils Vitamin E—as in Vitamin A Vitamin K is found in egg yolk, liver, wheat grain, soya beans		
MINERALS—calcium, iron, potassium and sodium, zinc, iodine, fluoride		Iron—lean red meat, whole grains, eggs Calcium—all dairy foods, bones of tinned fish Zinc—whole grains, eggs, meat, beans, milk Iodine—fish and all food grown in soils near the sea Fluoride is now added to most water supplies in Australia	Children should gain all their mineral requirements from food. Supplements should be given only on medical advice	Too little iron leads to low haemoglobin which carries oxygen in the blood around the body. The child will be pale and listless Too little calcium hinders bone and teeth growth Iodine deficiency can lead to intellectual disability Inadequate fluoride allows dental decay to occur

Table 7.2. Food groups

Food groups	Foods	Amounts needed
Group 1	Milk and cheese, which contain calcium, Vitamin B2 and animal protein	Young children need 600–900 ml of milk or milk products (yoghurt, custard) per day. 30 gm of cheese is equivalent to 1 glass milk
Group 2	Meat, fish and eggs, which are high in animal protein, iron and Vitamins B1, B2, B3	Meat includes beef, pork, lamb and chicken. Fish can be fresh, frozen or canned. The soft bones in canned fish also contain calcium. Eggs can be served any way, though preferably not fried. Dried peas, beans and lentils are high in vegetable protein but not in Vitamin B or iron Children need about 50 grams of meat or equivalent a day. One egg is equivalent to 25 grams of meat and half a cup of cooked peas, beans or lentils is equivalent to 45–50 grams of meat. Toddlers often are unable to eat enough to ensure adequate protein from vegetables alone
Group 3	Fruit and vegetables, which contain carbohydrates, fibre, vitamins and minerals	Young children need each day: one serving of a fruit high in Vitamin C—citrus, berries, tomato; one serving of a dark green leafy or yellow/orange vegetable and 2–3 servings of other fruit and vegetables
Group 4	Whole grain bread and cereals, which are the best source of complex carbohydrates. There are more vitamins in whole grain cereal, as well as necessary fibre	Children need 4–5 servings of this group each day. Cereals should not contain added sugar and bread should be served without jam or other sweet toppings
Group 5	Butter, margarine and oils, which contain fat and are needed to utilise fat soluble vitamins	Children should have 15–20 grams of fat a day. This includes that contained in foods as well as that added to breads

Water should be available for children all the time

The healthy diet pyramid

The pyramid was developed by the Australian Nutrition Foundation (1982). It shows the groups of foods that should be eaten most, those that can be eaten in moderation and those that should be eaten least. These foods should be prepared or cooked with no added fats, sugars or salt.

Eat most

The broad base of the pyramid indicates the foods that should make up the largest part of a healthy diet. These foods deliver mainly complex carbohydrates, and include:

- Cereals of all kinds and in all forms such as rice, barley, pasta, noodles, breakfast cereal (without added sugar).

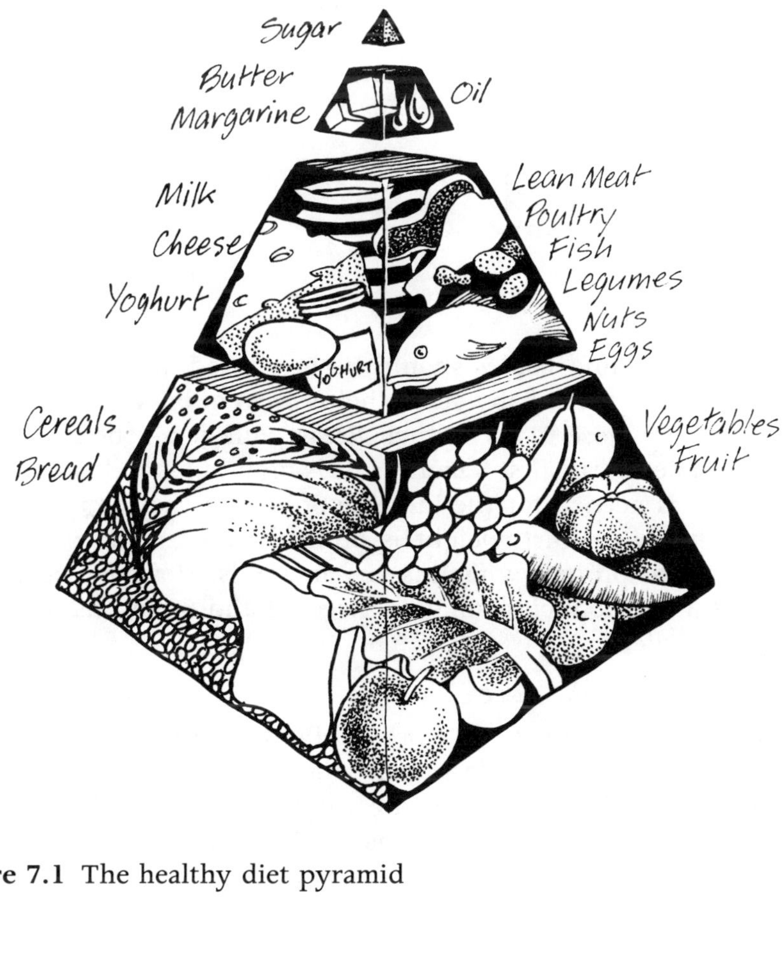

Figure 7.1 The healthy diet pyramid

- Bread of all forms, but especially bread and bread products made from whole grain cereal—including pitta bread, rye bread, muffins, damper and naan.
- All fruits and vegetables.

Eat moderately

This group includes foods high in protein.

- All meat (which should be lean), including poultry and fish as well as eggs.
- Dairy foods such as milk, cheese, yoghurt.
- Vegetables such as legumes (beans) and nuts.

Eat least

These foods are all high in sugar or fat and very small amounts should be eaten.

- Sugar (which is generally added to food during cooking, or stirred into tea, coffee, etc.)
- Fats such as butter and margarine.
- Any of the oils.

Children and food

0–1 year

Breast milk

Where possible young babies should be breast fed, as this is the best food nutritionally for the baby. It also helps prevent infection and brings mother and baby close to each other. Breast milk is all the food that is needed by babies in the first 6 months. It is high in fat and lactose (milk sugar), which is needed for the increase of weight that happens in the first 6 months, when birthweight is often doubled, and contains the right amounts of protein, vitamins and minerals. However, it is often advised to start introducing solids between 4 and 6 months to supplement the milk diet.

Breastfeeding and child care

Mothers frequently return to work while still wanting to maintain breastfeeding. Child-care professionals who encourage and make it easy for mothers to continue breastfeeding are helping to provide a healthy nutritional start for these babies, as well as giving support to the families.

Jennifer is in her early thirties and works as a clerical assistant in a busy city office. She has just returned to work after maternity leave and her son Alex is 6 months old. Alex is going to a child-care centre on the edge of the city. Jennifer wanted to continue breastfeeding as she thinks it is best for Alex and she enjoys the closeness it brings.

Jennifer chatted for a long time to the staff in the babies' room at the centre when she was finalising arrangements for Alex to come (she had him booked in since she was pregnant). The staff were very positive about her breastfeeding requests and said that several other mothers were successfully working and breastfeeding. The centre recently had an in-service course on maintaining breastfeeding from the Nursing Mothers' Association of Australia, so the staff were very keen to help mothers.

The child-care centre has a corner of the babies' room with easy chairs that are comfortable for breastfeeding. It is not totally isolated but it is peaceful, with pictures on the wall and attractive curtains at the window. This makes it an ideal place to breast feed Alex. He needs to be slightly away from all the action because at 6 months he can easily be distracted by other activities and stop feeding while he looks around.

Jennifer has a routine which now is working well, though it took a little while to get used to it and she was grateful for the encouragement of the child-care staff at this time. She has an efficient breast pump and expresses milk each day for freezing in special clearly labelled packs, which she takes to the child-care centre. Expressing milk makes her secrete more and she always has plenty. She wakes early in the morning and immediately feeds Alex, who has generally slept for 6–8 hours overnight. She then prepares herself and Alex for work and her partner makes the breakfast, which she takes time to eat before going off to the child-care centre.

After greeting the staff at the centre, Jennifer stores her expressed milk in the freezer and gives Alex another feed from the breast. There is sometimes another mother there feeding her baby as well. Alex isn't too hungry at this time, but a top-up now keeps him going until late morning when he has a little cereal and a bottle of expressed milk.

The staff at the centre know that Jennifer has spent time expressing her breast milk and they respect this by taking care of Alex's feeds, by ensuring that the milk is put into sterile bottles and warmed to the correct

Continued

temperature, which is tested before the bottle is given to Alex. As far as possible the same staff member feeds Alex and sits with him in the same chairs as his mother, holding him close as he is given the bottle. There is eye contact and a gentle stroking and skin contact.

Alex has also just started some baby cereal, which is given with the breast milk at the late morning feed. He generally has a small drink of breast milk or diluted unsweetened orange juice mid afternoon and then Jennifer breast feeds him again as soon as she gets to the centre in the late afternoon, before she and Alex go home.

The child-care centre staff always note in writing what each baby has drunk and eaten while at the centre, so Jennifer can see how much milk, cereal and orange juice Alex has had during the day.

A special note

The NHMRC guidelines on storing expressed milk indicate that breast milk can be stored in a refrigerator for 24 hours, in a freezer compartment of a single-door refrigerator for one month and for up to 3 months in a deep freeze.

Breast milk that has been warmed and not drunk should be discarded and never put back in the refrigerator for re-use. Warm milk is an ideal place for germs to grow; they will not be destroyed by refrigeration, and will grow again quickly when next removed from the refrigerator.

Formula feeding

The current recommendation is that babies under the age of 12 months should never be given cow's milk, but a formula milk which has been made especially for babies. Some nutritionists might even say that formula milk should be continued until over 12 months. In practice, most babies start to tolerate different proteins after 9 months of age as their diet becomes more varied, and their digestive systems can cope with cow's milk from then. The usual formulae are made from modified cow's milk and there are many brands on the market.

There are several important points regarding artificial feeding:

Sterility of all feeding equipment

The immune system of a young baby is still very immature and the risk of introduced infections is high. Contaminated feeding equipment can lead to severe diarrhoeal illness in infants. It is therefore important that all germs be killed by sterilising feeding equipment and anything, such as a dummy, that goes into a baby's mouth.

The most common way of sterilising feeding equipment is to use a sterilising solution. There are many of these commercial preparations available. Another simple way of sterilising is to boil all feeding utensils for 10 minutes.

Whatever the method of sterilisation, feeding equipment must be prepared in the same way:

- All dirty utensils must first be scrubbed, ensuring that all surfaces are clean. Left-over milk in one of the crevices of the bottle will still grow germs, even if put into a sterilising solution. Teats should be turned inside out and rubbed to clean old milk away from the hole. A bottle-brush should be used to get into any crevices on the feeding equipment.
- All articles should be rinsed after cleaning.
- Hands should be washed before coming into contact with the sterilising solution.
- All articles should be put into sterilising solution or water to be boiled, ensuring that each surface is in contact with the solution. There should be no air bubbles in the bottles, and it may be necessary to weigh down articles such as teats, which tend to float. Commercial sterilising kits often contain a utensil for pushing articles under the solution.
- The articles should be left in the solution for the correct amount of time—usually one hour for a commercial preparation, though the instructions for the specific product should be followed—and 10 minutes while the water is boiling if this method is being used. The time must be taken from the time the last article is placed in the solution.
- Care must be taken not to contaminate articles after sterilisation. Hands should be washed before handling any articles and only the outside of bottles and bottle discs should be touched. It is best to

use tongs for handing teats, though care should be taken if using a commercial solution that the tongs will not react with the solution. Plastic (not metal) tongs need to be used with some solutions.
- Commercial sterilising solutions should be changed according to the instructions, which is usually every 24 hours.

At about 8+ months of age a baby will start crawling around the floor. At this stage, in a home or family day-care situation, ensuring that feeding utensils are scrubbed, rinsed and kept scrupulously clean is usually all that is needed. It seems rather ironic to have the baby crawling around the floor under the table on which the mother is sterilising feeding utensils!

Sterilisation of feeding equipment should continue past the crawling age in large group care, as there is the added hazard of germs from other children. A general rule would be to sterilise until the child is using a cup.

Making up the formula

This must be done exactly to instructions, as the baby's nutritional intake depends upon the strength of the formula being correct. A formula that is too weak will mean the baby will be hungry and not grow as he should. A formula that is too strong can cause digestive upsets and obesity.

Most parents get advice about formula feeding from the community child-health nurse and feel confident about making up the feeds. Most parents coming to a child-care setting bring bottles that are already made up, but it is important that child-care professionals should follow the given instructions if feeds need to made up in care.

Bottles that have been prepared at home need to be kept cold en route to child care and refrigerated immediately on arrival. If the parents cannot keep the bottles cool, then it best if the formula is made up in child care so that any risk of contamination is eliminated.

A few points when making up the formula:

- The surface where the formula will be made should be clean and clear.
- All equipment must be ready, including cooled boiled water in a closed container.
- Hands must be well washed before commencing to make up the formula.
- The exact measure of cooled boiled water should be placed in the bottles. The boiled water should be cooled because vitamins in the formula are destroyed if the water is hot.

- The correct amount of powder or liquid formula should be added to the water in the bottles. The measurements for powder often require a flat measure, and a sterile plastic knife is usually used. A measuring scoop is provided with powdered formula.
- Teats, discs and bottle tops are put into place so that the milk is covered; it is then immediately put into the refrigerator until ready for use.

Bottle-feeding the baby

There should be minimal difference between breastfeeding and bottle feeding the baby. Nutritional requirements should certainly be met, but so should emotional needs. Feeding time is a time for carer and baby, and belongs to no one else. There should be as few interruptions as possible.

Items for feeding should be prepared before picking up the baby, though hungry babies can become distressed very quickly and should be comforted. Hands should be washed and the bottle taken out of the refrigerator to be warmed. Most babies prefer feeds at body temperature. This should be done by standing the covered bottle in a container of hot water and then uncovering the bottle, gently shaking to ensure even distribution of heat, and then testing the heat by dropping some milk onto the tender part of the inside of the arm. Microwaves should not be used for heating bottles as the heat distribution is often very uneven and there can be cold parts of the formula and parts that are so hot that a baby's mouth could be badly burned.

Teat holes should be the right size for each baby. Young babies need smaller holes than do older babies, but holes that are too small will mean that babies do not get enough milk and give up before they have had enough. This means they do not settle easily in the short term and may have growth problems in the long term. A general rule even for a young baby is that the milk should drip from the teat at the rate of one drop per second and get faster as the baby gets older, though this depends on the type of teat.

Caregiver and baby should sit together in a comfortable, relaxed and attractive place. The baby should be held close to the caregiver's body and the bottle tipped so that milk fills the teat. The tilt of the bottle and the level of the fluid should continually be checked to ensure that the baby is not sucking in air. Some babies will suck hard and long until the bottle is finished or until they have had enough. Other babies will suck for a while and then want a rest. Each baby's personality needs to be taken into account. This is a time for eye contact, for stroking, perhaps for gentle, quiet reassuring talk.

Most babies do get some wind during bottle feeding and need to be sat up straight and be burped to expel wind which otherwise might cause pain. Some gentle back rubbing is often done at this time too. It is a good idea to have a bib or other cloth to wipe up any of the feed that comes up with the wind. Any unused formula should be immediately discarded.

Babies should never be left alone with a bottle propped on a pillow. Apart from the danger of choking, the baby is getting no emotional support or contact with another person, which is an important part of feeding.

Starting solids

Starting solids goes together with getting teeth (though first foods do not need teeth for chewing). Babies will have developed control over the muscles in the jaw and co-ordination with swallowing. The digestive system is also more mature. Babies generally do not need any food other than milk for the first 6 months. Some parents and caregivers wonder about giving orange or other juices. This is not necessary, as there is enough vitamin C in breast milk and formula, but juices such as orange, apple or prune diluted with 1 part juice and 2 parts water may be given after 3–4 months of age. The juice should be pure juice that has no added sugar and is diluted with cool boiled water. Care should be taken to make sure that the baby still gets the right amount of breast or formula feeds.

First solids

Modified cereals mixed with breast milk or formula are usually the first solid foods given to babies. Rice cereals are often used, as there is very little allergy to these and they are easily digested. Most baby cereals are fortified with iron because, from around 6 months of age, babies will not get enough iron from milk alone.

Other first foods are cooked fruit such as apple, and vegetables such as pumpkin, potato, broccoli, zucchini or carrot that have been pureed, and soft fresh fruit such as well mashed banana. It is a good idea to try only one new food at a time for a few days in case the baby is allergic to the new food. It will then be easy to recognise which food might cause the reaction. Fresh food should be used where possible, and no sugar or salt added to the cooking.

Eggs are not usually given until after 7 months of age because of the risk of allergy. A good idea is to give the baby a small taste of egg yolk initially and then slowly increase the amount over a period of time. The same pattern can be followed with egg white.

By the time the baby is 8–9 months old, other textures and tastes will be offered. Lumpier cereal can now be introduced, as can mashed rather than pureed fruit and vegetables so that the texture is firmer. Lumpier food is also good for baby finger-, or should we say fist-, food!

It is important that babies are given the chance to recognise individual foods. As far as possible, the foods should be kept separate on the same plate so that babies can start to recognise different tastes, textures and colours. Often babies are given all vegetables mixed up together, where there is no chance of identifying anything. Many parents and child-care centres freeze individual servings of single vegetables in ice cube trays so there is a ready supply. Freezing maintains taste, texture and the nutrients. Reheating can destroy vitamins, but this can be reduced by using a microwave at low power to reheat the vegetables. The vegetables need to be stirred to ensure even distribution of heat.

At 12 months many babies are usually enjoying the family meal, which has been modified by mashing vegetables and chopping or mincing meat finely. Hard raw foods such as apples and carrots, which could cause choking, should all be grated.

Fresh or commercially prepared baby foods

Many parents and some children's services wonder about the best type of food for infants. The older style of baby food in tins or jars had added sugar and salt. Babies often developed a taste for the sugar and salt, which made them less responsive to freshly cooked foods that did not contain the additives. Market pressures due to parental demand have caused commercial baby foods with no added sugar and salt to become easily available. There will be some additives in the form of emulsifiers, but these are not harmful.

Nutritionally the commercially prepared foods are adequate. Where they fall down is in the lack of texture and taste and in attractive presentation. Most adults faced with the choice of a home-cooked meal made with fresh ingredients or a can of stew and vegetables (which is quite nutritionally sound) would choose the freshly cooked meal without hesitation. The taste is far preferable, there is a wider range of textures and it looks much more attractive and appetising. Babies need to have the same benefits as adults and they also need a variety of food.

There is no doubt that there are times, such as travelling, when it is useful to use commercially prepared food, but it is more interesting for the baby if it is not used on a daily or even regular basis.

Giving solids

Babies react to first solids in different ways. Some immediately know what to do with this new texture and taste and happily swallow, others screw up their faces and let the new substance drip out of their mouth.

A spoon going into the mouth is also a new experience and, with newly developed eye-hand coordination, it is an exciting new toy to grab. Sometimes the first solid foods are given while holding the baby on a lap. This soon becomes very difficult as the baby is reaching out, grabbing the spoon while the caregiver is aiming for the mouth. A suitable feeding chair makes mealtime a much more enjoyable experience and babies are usually able to sit at 6+ months of age. Remember that all children need to have safety harnesses used in any form of feeding chair, whether high or low.

Mealtimes should be happy times, where both babies and caregivers are relaxed. This reinforces the positive experience relating to nutritious food. Feeding is likely to be messy, but this will not be a problem if a covering is put on the floor under the chair or if the chair is placed on a floor that is easily cleaned. Bibs or other coverings to protect clothes may also be needed. It is often useful to have two spoons, one for the baby and one for the feeder. Babies learn about their world by movement and by sensory experience. The baby of 6+ months baby will feel the food (so make sure her hands have first been washed), will get some into her mouth with her fingers and maybe some into her hair; she will then pick up the spoon, perhaps first banging it on the tray surface, before putting the spoon into the food, turning it over, and aiming for her mouth.

It is important that babies are given the opportunity to feed themselves, but care does need to be taken that some of the food has actually been eaten rather than spread on the face or fallen on the floor. Leaving an 8–9-month-old baby with a plate of mashed vegetables and a spoon may result in very little being eaten. Babies of this age usually still need some assistance with feeding, and they certainly need the reassurance of a responsive adult during mealtime. Finger food such as strips of bread or toast and grated cheese or apple are easier for baby to handle and can be managed alone, though there still needs to be emotional and social support given.

Continuing with milk

Milk (and milk products) should remain part of a baby's diet even when nutrients are being obtained from solid food. Milk remains a good source of protein and calcium and a baby 6–12 months of age would generally have a bottle of milk or a breast feed after each meal. Some babies of this age, especially those being breast fed, like a last suckle during the evening. Bottles in bed, when babies are able to hold their bottle, may be comforting but are not advisable due to the danger of choking, and because the lactose in the milk may decay the teeth.

Helena is 9 months old and has been coming to this family day care home for 4 months. Both her parents came from Greece when they were small children. Helena has just been weaned and is now having formula from a bottle. Her mother tried to give her a feeding cup but, although she accepts this for juice, she prefers to take milk from a bottle.

Helena wakes very early in the morning and is given a bottle of formula that was made up the previous evening. Her mother gets herself ready for the day and Helena has breakfast with her parents. Helena sits in a high chair at the table and has half a Weetbix made soft with warm formula, a thin, small slice of smooth wholemeal toast with a smear of peanut butter and a small feeding cup of orange juice. She needs some assistance to eat the Weetbix but she feeds herself the toast, dropping a small bit on the floor. She again needs some help with the feeding cup as she is still learning to tip it up. When she is finished with the cup she throws it on the floor and looks to see where it has gone.

Helena's father cleans up and they then go to child care, where she is greeted by her caregiver and two other children aged 3 and 4. They are almost ready to take the 4-year-old to pre-school.

Helena is happy in the pusher as she goes off with her caregiver and the other children. On their return she crawls around, exploring her play area and sucking on her toys, until about 10 o'clock when she has some grated apple and a small drink of formula from a bottle. She feeds herself the apple and has her bottle on her caregiver's lap. She then settles happily in her cot and sleeps until about noon, when it is time to go to pre-school to collect the older child.

Lunch is ready when they get back and everyone washes their hands. Helena has some minced lamb with small amounts of mashed potato, pumpkin and broccoli. Helena eats most of this by herself, with both spoon and fingers, as she sits up in her chair at the table with the others. The other children also have the same meal, though the lamb is sliced rather that minced and their vegetables are not mashed, apart from the potatoes, which they prefer this way. For dessert all children have plain unsweetened yoghurt with sliced banana for the older children and mashed banana for Helena.

Helena has another sleep in the afternoon, having had a bottle of formula before settling. She had her bottle in the caregiver's lap, though she half held the bottle herself. After she wakes, late afternoon tea is a small drink of diluted apple and blackcurrant juice and a homemade rusk with a smear of Vegemite. She is happily playing on the floor beside the other children when her father arrives to pick her up at 4.30 pm.

The evening meal for Helena is some coddled egg and mashed spinach with a sliver of toast, and after another bottle of formula she is soon asleep.

1–2 years

This is the time of exploration, when the world becomes available to the now mobile child. Toddlers do not need to be taken to interesting places in the house or in the child-care centre, they can now move and get there themselves. All of this becomes so interesting that food may be forgotten at times. Toddlers are learning how to exert their rights and they have likes and dislikes for lots of things, including toys, clothes and food.

The growth rate of children slows somewhat in the second year but there is an increased level of activity once the child is running around.

Snacks

Toddlers sometimes find it difficult to last from one meal to the next and they tend to graze (this term is one I have used for many years, and is also used by Stanton, 1990). They play and then want a snack to keep them going over the next period. Toddlers seem to exist on snacks and some caregivers and parents despair that they will ever eat a full meal.

For toddlers, snacks constitute a meal. The toddler who is thirsty at 11am and is given fruit juice or milk is not going to eat lunch half an hour later. The drink was a meal. The toddler who is given nothing when thirsty at 11am is going to be so tired and distressed by lunchtime that she won't be able to eat all her meal and will wake up from her afternoon sleep hungry and miserable.

This can become a real nutritional problem when sweet biscuits, crisps and other unsuitable foods are given to children between meals. This means that proper meals will not be eaten and the main food for the day is made up of food that does not provide the required nutritional requirements for a growing child.

The nutritional problem is solved if snacks are made up only of nutritious food such as a piece of fruit, a slice of cheese, a glass of milk, a piece of bread with peanut butter or Vegemite. However, this does not address the problem of how to encourage toddlers to settle into routines of eating main meals with small snacks in between.

Routines

Child-care routines need to be very sympathetic to both the developmental and nutritional needs of toddlers as they move through this second year, which marks the transition from infant to young child. Toddlers may not be able to fit in easily with the general feeding routines planned for the service and may need to have an individual routine until they settle into more established feeding patterns. At the same time the toddler needs to be gently encouraged to settle into these established feeding patterns, as it is important nutritionally as well as socially for them to do this.

Paul is 18 months old and walking and running well. He enjoys climbing on the outdoor equipment and is an active child. He has been in child care for the last 6 months, so is well used to the staff and the environment.

Paul's parents need to start work very early and they find the mornings are becoming difficult as Paul is sleeping later, is naturally grumpy when woken, and likes to take his time getting dressed. There is no way he can be hurried over his breakfast and there have been a couple of occasions when he cried and did not eat his breakfast.

His parents discuss the situation with the child-care staff and decide it would be best for Paul to have his breakfast at the centre so that he can take his time and eat in an unhurried way. The centre provides breakfast for an extra charge each week.

Paul's routine now goes like this:

Paul is left to sleep while his parents have their own breakfast. He has a glass of milk when he awakes, is given a wash and tries to dress himself, though his parents need to give lots of assistance. His parents also get ready for work. They then leave for child care about 15 minutes earlier than they had done in the past.

On arrival at child care, Paul and his parents wash their hands and sit down at the table set up for breakfast in a light and bright part of the centre. His parents stay chatting with him and sometimes have a piece of fruit, too, while he eats his breakfast. Paul has some unsweetened whole grain cereal and cow's milk with chopped fresh fruit and a small dollop of yoghurt on top. He enjoys this and engages with his parents and the other children as he eats. Toast is offered or some other form of bread, such as muffins or pitta bread, with margarine, Vegemite, peanut butter or tofu. Unsweetened diluted fruit juice is available. Paul's parents enjoy this time with him over breakfast and they get to know the other children, parents and staff much more than they had in the past. It doesn't matter if Paul has not finished breakfast before they need to leave. He can take his time while they go off to work, having had a good start to the day.

Continued

The child-care staff observe the children carefully and can tell which child might be restless because of tiredness or hunger. They have certain periods for snacks and meals, but they are extended periods. Paul has a fairly early breakfast, so he is one of the first children to have his snack. Other children have their snack a little later. The staff find the routine works well. Children in their second year still need assistance with hand washing and sitting at the table, and having the children come in gradually helps the staff to give the individual attention each child needs.

Paul washes his hands before morning tea and sits at the table with one or two other children. There are platters of fruit containing apples, pears or bananas (the fruit varies and sometimes it is dried fruit and cheese). Many of the children are still unable to name the foods but can happily indicate which fruits they want. The fruit is handed to the children by the staff, using tongs, as the children's hands will touch their mouths. A small glass of milk is offered to each child. Each child puts his cup and plate on the trolley when finished. Any fruit scraps are put into a small bucket and the children help give these to the pet guinea pig later in the day.

Lunch is prepared so that it is ready before the first child starts getting tired. Food is always served by staff at the table. Paul again is one of the first to wash his hands and get ready for lunch. A caregiver is ready for him as he sits down and chats to him about what is for lunch. Today it is tomato, spinach, cheese and potato slice and salad made from lettuce, grated carrot and cold cooked broccoli. The caregiver has noticed that Paul ate lots of fruit at morning tea so he is not surprised when Paul doesn't quite finish his first helping. Paul has a teaspoon with which to eat, but he also uses his fingers, and there is often some finger food provided for this group. Water is poured into stable cups which do not tip over easily but which the children can handle easily. As they get older they will pour their own drinks from small jugs.

Paul has only a very small second course. This child-care centre as far as possible serves a dessert that has no added sugar, though occasionally a little honey is used. This means that a child who has not eaten all the first course will still have a nutritious second course. It might be fruit that is served fresh, either whole or chopped into a fruit salad. Sometimes, if the fruit is naturally sweet, it will be stewed and perhaps served with light cream cheese or frozen yoghurt; at other times a cereal pudding such as rice or tapioca sweetened with fruit is served and is very popular with the children.

Continued

The children all put their plates and cutlery on the trolley again after lunch. By now Paul is very tired and the caregiver quickly settles him for a sleep.

Paul sleeps for more than 2 hours and on waking is still drowsy, so slowly dresses with assistance, washes his hands and is offered a snack of wholegrain bread with toppings of avocado and light cream cheese. Paul is thirsty and refuses the food but drinks a glass of milk instead. He feels more awake then and goes off to play outdoors. He is offered the snack later in the afternoon just before his mother is due to pick him up. He now eats it hungrily with a small glass of fruit juice.

It is around 4pm when Paul's mother arrives and they head off to the supermarket together. This is usually an enjoyable time as they can share getting things off the shelves where possible. The worst time is the check-out, where there are lots of sweets displayed. Paul starts pointing longingly but his mother has now had lots of practice at this and distracts him away from the sweets by getting him to help unload the trolley.

At home Paul often has some grated apple or a few grapes, as dinner is usually not until 6.30 pm. This is the only meal of the day that the family eat at home together and they value this time. The food is usually simple and complements what Paul has had during the day. Tonight they have Chinese noodles and stir-fried chicken and vegetables. Paul has a glass of milk to follow. He then cleans his teeth, has a cuddle, a bedtime story and a kiss and, after a couple of times getting out of bed and calling to his parents, he falls fast asleep.

Milk

Milk and milk products are still important in the diet of a toddler and they should have 600 ml per day of milk. This includes milk products such as yoghurt or cheese, but an increasing amount of the toddler's nutritional needs should be gained from other foods. A glass of milk should be offered as a snack and at some meals, but protein and calcium should also be obtained from cheese, eggs, yoghurt, fish and meat.

Fruit juice

Unsweetened fruit juice is a good source of carbohydrates, vitamins and minerals. It does not provide any fibre, so whole fruit should also be eaten. It is a good idea to give toddlers only small amounts of diluted fruit juice and ensure that there is enough whole fruit in their diet.

There is sometimes a problem with apple juice and it is thought that perhaps it might be the cause of bouts of non-infective diarrhoea in toddlers.

Water

Toddlers should also be offered plain water and this should be available at all times, especially in the warmer weather. Adults also should drink plain water when thirsty rather than carbonated sweet drinks.

2–5 years

This is a time of consolidation where all the huge developmental leaps of the first 2 years are built upon. Language development goes ahead by leaps and bounds and the child increasingly will recognise and ask for specific types of food. The level of motor coordination is such that the child becomes able to use a knife and fork for cutting food. Socially, he enjoys the responsibility of getting the table ready for lunch and of helping serve the meal. The presence of the chewing molars means that most foods can now be eaten, though extreme care should still be taken with whole nuts until the child is older than 4–5 years.

Personal preferences for food may become more pronounced. Many children are very definite about their likes and dislikes and are sometimes loath to try new food. A friendly environment where nutritious food is attractively served and new foods are encouraged will help the child develop positive eating habits.

Working with parents continues to be very important, and now is the time when the influence of both child care and home is challenged by television and other forms of advertising for inappropriate foods and by the easy availability of non-nutritious foods in supermarkets and other stores. Fast food chains beckon and even give gifts in order to bribe children into cajoling their parents to eat or buy food at their store.

Almeido is 4 years old and lives with his mother, who is a high school teacher. She and Almeido came to Australia from Chile two years ago. Almeido's parents are separated and his father still lives in Chile, though he and his mother have many other relatives in Australia.

Almeido's mother usually has to wake him each morning and he washes and dresses himself before coming out for breakfast. There is

Continued

always muesli and fresh fruit with milk, and sometimes he also has toast. He would rather like some other sort of breakfast cereal which is sweeter (he's seen it in the supermarket) but his mother just says 'no' and explains it has too much sugar in it. Sometimes at weekends he is allowed to have some jam on his toast or raisin bread. His mother says jam is 'treat food' and she smiles at him when she says it. Sometimes, too, he has sweet desserts at one of his relative's homes but he knows that this is also treat food.

Almeido is an active, healthy child who enjoys the child-care centre he attends. He rushes in every day, greeting the staff and other children, and is busy with a variety of activities until morning tea time. He helps pack up the tables that are needed for morning tea and wipes them over before going to wash his hands. Morning tea comes on a trolley and Almeido happily places platters of fresh and dried fruit and individual bowls on each table. Individual jugs of milk are also placed on each table and the children pour their own.

Everyone chatters happily over morning tea and the staff sit sharing the conversation. Today they are going to dig in the vegetable garden and plant some spinach and tomatoes, so there is lots to talk about. Yesterday some of the children went to the plant nursery down the road and chose the seedlings to plant. The woman in the nursery told them how she grew them from seeds and gave them some seeds to put in a pot.

After morning tea they sit on the mat together having a story about the Great Big Enormous Turnip (see Books for children). Almeido tells the teacher that he doesn't think the spinach will grow that big, and everyone agrees. But they discuss how hard it was to pull up the turnip. They then go out to the garden and everyone is very busy digging, raking, watering and planting right up to lunch.

Almeido especially liked poking holes in the damp earth and putting the plants in. He is looking forward to them growing, and especially having spinach pie with cheese and tomato on top.

Everyone's hands are washed before lunch and a couple of children need to change their t-shirts too. Before they went to the table for lunch they listened to a funny song about a girl called Leanne who thought she didn't like vegetables but then found out she did (ABC 1994).

Lunch today is a smorgasbord of salads, meats, cheese and breads. It is set out on a table so that the children can take what they prefer. The cook has made it look really attractive, which makes Almeido even

Continued

hungrier and he uses tongs to take some pitta bread, some tomatoes, some grated carrot, some cucumber, a piece of cheese and a chicken drumstick and then sits down with his friends to eat it. The table has a bright flowery cloth on it and some of the other children had picked some flowers when they were in the garden and they put them in a vase on the table. One of the child-care students thought it looked a bit like a restaurant and was amazed at how all the children enjoyed their food and chatted throughout the meal.

Almeido had second helpings. There was a platter of apples and pears for anyone who wanted something else and Almeido did have a slice of pear. There was water to drink.

The children all helped clear up from lunch and then they went to have a rest. Almeido often doesn't sleep after lunch but he likes looking at the stories and the pictures in books. He has one today that he chose from the library when the older children went to get books a couple of days ago. It is all about farms and the food the farmers grow and the animals that give food too. Almeido decides he will make a farm with the blocks and toy animals after rest time.

Afternoon tea is some home-made guacamole dip with sliced vegetables and water biscuits, with a glass of fruit juice. Almeido's mother is late coming today as she has a staff meeting, so he has a glass of milk before going home about 5.30 pm, though not before he shows her the garden they have planted.

They call in on Almeido's cousin and aunt on the way home. The children there have some crisps and Almeido is given some—'only a few' his mother says. Then it is home where his mother gets out the paella she made last night. Almeido loves the rice and fish and eats with his mother, telling her about the farm he made at child care. He was a bit sad when he had to pack it up before he went home. He shares a banana and yoghurt with his mother before he cleans his teeth and chooses a story for bedtime.

5–12 year olds

This age group now is having to cope with making independent choices about food. They are sometimes in such a rush that they miss breakfast and make up with non-nutritious snacks at morning break time. Lunch is often a cut lunch from home and the nutritional value of this is dependent on many factors, including parental knowledge, education, income level and household organisation.

Other children purchase lunch from the school canteen. Many school canteens are now providing more nutritious foods but there are still others who rely on the canteen for funds or who have contracted the canteen out to private profit-making enterprises. Nutrition comes a poor second to profit in these situations. So there are still many canteens selling foods that are far too high in fat and sugar and far too low in complex carbohydrates, protein, vitamins and minerals.

Out of school hours child care can partly solve the breakfast problem by providing a nutritious breakfast for those children who have not eaten. There can be a charge for this, or the breakfast program might be subsidised in some way by a local service organisation. The breakfast can be relatively simple to prepare if it is cereal, milk and toast. This has the added advantage of providing a social activity as well. The snacks provided after school should be made up of fruit and raw vegetables plus breads with nutritious yet inexpensive toppings such as Vegemite, cheese, tofu or peanut butter, and water to drink.

One of the other concerns, especially with girls, as adolescence approaches is the beginning of eating disorders. Encouraging all children to feel good about themselves can perhaps lessen the dissatisfaction many girls feel about their bodies, though the cause of eating disorders is much more complex than self-esteem alone. Adolescent girls also need an adequate intake of iron to cope with the loss of blood (which contains iron) when menstruation starts.

Amelia is 9 years old and attends the local primary school, where she is in Year 4. She is usually one of the first up at home in the morning and gets herself a glass of orange juice before she starts setting the table for breakfast. The family try as much as possible to have breakfast together, though this frequently doesn't work because Amelia's mother often has early meetings. When this happens, her father is kept busy packing snacks and lunches for Amelia and her two older brothers, though they do all help him with this.

Amelia sometimes wishes she could buy her lunch or recess snack from the school canteen more often, but her parents are very particular about what she eats. Every week or so she is given money for the canteen but other days she takes her snack and lunch from home.

The food in the lunch box is always varied. Amelia gets very tired of sandwiches and her parents understand this. At weekends they take it in

Continued

turn to shop and Amelia often goes too and chooses food for her lunches. Her mother worries about putting meat in the lunch box in the warm weather in case it becomes contaminated by germs, so she is pleased when Amelia chooses to take crunchy salad vegetables like raw celery, carrot, cauliflower, beans, snow peas, sprouts, cherry tomatoes or capsicum, which she can eat with some cheese, nuts or a boiled egg.

There is usually some bread or a wholemeal roll that is lightly spread with margarine or cream cheese and which Amelia eats plain or fills with the salad vegetables or cheese. Sometimes Amelia surprises her parents and asks for a plain peanut butter sandwich, to which she adds some raisins. A piece of fruit such as an apple, a banana or orange is always there and this is varied with other fruits in season such as strawberries, melon, grapes or paw-paw though these sometimes get squashed in the lunch box, but Amelia can certainly have them at home.

At school, Amelia can choose what she would like for morning snack from the range of foods in her lunch box. She usually has a drink of water, too. Her lunch is eaten with friends under the trees in the school yard. The group of children do sometimes swap food, though many of the lunches are similar. The class teacher recently had a visiting nutritionist to talk to the class and he invited the parents along too. There was lots of printed material about children and nutrition available for those parents who couldn't make it. There is a huge poster of the 'Healthy Diet Pyramid' on the wall with pictures of the different foods in each section. Many of the children now ask their parents for whole grain bread and salad fillings for lunch time.

Menu planning and food preparation

Parental involvement

Food preferences should be discussed with parents on enrolment, as well as the nutrition policy of the service. There will be many differences in food preferences between individual children and families and between ethnic groups and cultures. This gives an ideal opportunity to plan eating experiences for children by introducing new foods. Any food allergies must be carefully noted on enrolment and the menu planned to keep that child free of those foods.

Parents need to know the ongoing menu, which can be given to them individually and/or placed on the door or notice board where it will be easily seen. This is important, not only to let parents know what their child has for meals, but so that they can plan their family meal times without too much repetition. Sometimes parents are happy to share popular family recipes, which also adds variety to the menu.

Nutritional needs

Planning an ongoing menu is generally the responsibility of several staff, and parents are encouraged to have input as well as listening to the ideas of the children. Some services also seek advice from a community dietitian or nutritionist in order to ensure that the menu is nutritionally sound.

There should be a variety of foods, which can be checked for adequate daily quantities and variety with the healthy diet pyramid as well as the basic five food groups. A variety of foods from within each category can be used so that children experience different types of fruit, vegetables, cereals, meats and other foods. A range of tastes, textures, colours, shapes and sizes also provides essential variety within the menu.

Foods used will depend on the season and economic availability of foods. Children will respond more to salads in summer and hot foods such as soup on a cold winter's day.

Food hygiene

This is a crucial part of preventing disease in child care. Micro-organisms grow very quickly in foods and food poisoning can kill children.

There are two main points to bear in mind regarding food hygiene:

1. That food is not contaminated when purchased
2. That food is not contaminated within the children's service

Purchasing food

All food should be checked for freshness and that it is within the 'use by' date. Where possible, food can be bought from wholesalers where the produce can be assessed. Supermarkets often drape fresh food in cling wrap, which may prevent people handling the food but also stops the purchaser assessing what is the state of the bottom layer of fruit or vegetables.

Storing food

- All perishable foods need to be stored in a refrigerator that is kept at a temperature under 4° Celsius. A thermometer should be kept in the fridge to enable kitchen staff to check the temperature.
- All food that is to be kept hot should be kept at a temperature above 60° Celsius.
- Any food that has not been kept hot or cold as required should be thrown out. A general rule is 'If in doubt, throw it out'.

- Cooked and uncooked foods should be stored separately. Micro-organisms from uncooked foods can otherwise contaminate cooked foods, which are then given directly to children.

Preparing food

- Staff who are responsible for changing nappies should not be involved in food preparation.
- The food preparation area and kitchen should be free of flies, other insects and vermin such as mice.
- All surfaces on which food is prepared should be non-porous and be able to be scrubbed.
- The food preparation area and kitchen should have a separate wash basin situated in the kitchen (apart from the sink) and soap for the kitchen staff to wash their hands easily. Disposable paper towels should be used.
- Separate utensils should be used when preparing cooked and uncooked food.
- Kitchen staff should wear protective clothing such as aprons and hair covering if the hair is long. The apron should not be worn out of the kitchen.

Serving food

- Food should be served on plain crockery that has no grooves or cracks in which micro-organisms can grow.
- All crockery and cutlery used should be able to withstand the high temperatures needed for washing. Ideally a dishwasher should be used after dishes are wiped clear of food.
- Food that has been brought from home must be heated to 60° Celsius, cooled down and immediately served. Food should not be merely heated to the temperature needed by the child, as this is the temperature that encourages the growth of micro-organisms.
- Food should be heated only once, and if not eaten should be thrown out.
- Any left-over food must be discarded.

(NHMRC 1997)

Some common concerns about food

Fresh, frozen, dried or canned?

Many people think that the nutritional value of frozen, dried or canned food is non-existent and that the only food worth eating is fresh.

Fresh food generally tastes more pleasing, looks more attractive and has a greater range of textures, and these are very important points when choosing food for children. Nutritional content, however, is scarcely altered by drying, canning or freezing, apart from fibre being eliminated if food such as vegetables and fruit have been peeled or cereal highly processed. Vitamin C contained in fresh food is unstable once the food is cooked, so raw fresh fruit and vegetables are a necessary part of any child or adult's diet.

Additives to food

Processed food often contains additives that are used to preserve food, to enhance colour and flavour, or to maintain the texture. Other additives such as salt, sugar and fat are often used to make the taste seem more appealing. More and more manufacturers are now producing foods with no added salt or sugar and fat, so the label should be checked before purchasing food.

Some of the chemicals used with processed foods also occur naturally in fresh foods. Salicylates, which are added to many processed foods, are also found in fresh fruit and vegetables. Fresh foods sometimes contain natural chemicals that are poisonous. Potatoes naturally contain a chemical called solanine, which is poisonous if eaten in large quantities.

Food allergy in children

Food allergy is a potentially serious condition in children and occurs as a result of an immune reaction to natural foods as well as some additives. Serious allergy to foods such as eggs, peanuts, mangoes, etc. can cause anaphylactic shock and death.

Other foods may cause urticarial skin rashes (hives), vomiting, asthma and other symptoms. Some allergies may be easily identified and the food totally eliminated from the diet. In other cases it is much harder to identify the cause of the reaction and the child would need many skin tests to see if there is a definite allergy to one or more particular foods (or substances contained in the foods).

Food sensitivity and children

Many parents observe behavioural changes such as hyperactivity in children which they feel sure are due to certain foods, and especially foods with red and yellow colouring. The biochemical links between the food and the behaviour are not yet fully established, although it is known that some children are sensitive to the chemicals in some foods.

It should also be remembered that children's behaviour changes for a variety of reasons, such as being bored, not having appropriate activities or during a period of developmental change.

What is known is that too much fast-acting sugar (as found in lollies and soft drinks of all colours) in one hit will cause the blood sugar to rise sharply, thus causing more insulin to be quickly made. This could certainly alter a child's behaviour. It is, however, very easy to prevent by ensuring that the child has a well balanced nutritional diet where the sugar needed by the body is obtained from fresh fruits, vegetables and cereals and that there is no fast consumption of high-sugar foods.

Elimination diets

These are time-consuming tests that go on over several weeks. All foods that are known to cause sensitivity (either by natural or added chemicals) are removed from the diet. The child still needs to have a well-balanced and nutritious diet, and for this reason the tests should only be carried out by a qualified dietitian or nutritionist.

If there is no change in the child's symptoms after several weeks, then a sensitivity to food is not the problem. If the symptoms disappear, then foods are slowly reintroduced to see if the food causing the sensitivity can be identified.

Lactose intolerance

Some children, especially those of Asian and Middle Eastern origin, are unable to tolerate the lactose in milk. This is due to their body stopping production of an enzyme called lactase, which is needed to digest lactose. This results in the lactose sitting undigested in the bowel, causing diarrhoea.

Tests can be carried out to confirm the absence of lactase. Children with lactose intolerance usually do not need to avoid foods such as butter or cheese as they contain very little lactose. Yoghurt is usually tolerated as the lactose has been broken down during the thickening process.

For these children, milk drinks need to be of a type that is lactose-free. There are some forms of cow's milk from which the lactose has been removed. Soya bean milk is also free of lactose. Calcium supplements will need to be taken if the soya bean milk does not have a calcium supplement.

'Treat' food

It is impossible to ignore the fact that children are surrounded by food that has little or no nutritional value, and it is difficult (unless a child has a disease such as diabetes) to prevent them having these foods at some time. These high-sugar, high-fat foods should be regarded as treats for very special occasions, rather than given on a regular basis. They certainly have no place as part of the regular menu in a child-care setting.

Fast foods, especially those served by restaurants designed to attract children, come into the 'treat food' category. The family nutritional status will not be compromised by having an occasional meal in such a place, but eating these meals frequently will not meet nutritional needs.

Nutrition education and children

Education about food is part of the nutrition program in any children's service. Young children will not understand the concepts of protein, carbohydrates or other food constituents but they can understand that some food is encouraged more than others. Many people describe food as 'good' or 'bad' food, which tends to place a moral connotation on food that is inappropriate. Some Aboriginal communities have got around this problem by dividing food into 'strong' and 'worry' food.

Attitudes toward food

Feelings and attitudes about food start forming when very young. A baby who is breast fed gets emotional warmth as well as nutrients. A baby who is bottle fed also needs that emotional warmth. A relaxed mother or caregiver sitting in a comfortable place gives the baby the message that the food and feeding time, as well as the baby, are important.

Poor food habits can also be developed early. Putting honey on a dummy or teat of a crying or restless baby encourages a taste for sweet things, as well as giving the baby the message that sweet things are pacifiers. This is the beginning of the dangerous nutritional habits of comforting a distressed child with sweet foods such as lollies and biscuits. This, in turn, may lead to adults who comfort themselves with gorging and eating too many sweet foods.

A toddler who is rushed at meals, or expected to wait for a meal, will have unpleasant experiences with food. Mealtimes should be enjoyable, relaxed times with warm friendly interactions between staff and children.

Older children need also to have happy experiences with food and mealtimes. Lunchtime is a great opportunity to sit and discuss what has happened during the morning, to reflect upon and reinforce experiences together over a happy meal. Discussing food over a meal also reinforces nutritional concepts. Adults choose to go out for meals with friends, or have meals with friends at home. It is part of our ongoing social development, and it is no different for children. Happy experiences at mealtimes, together with an interesting meal, help form very positive attitudes to food.

Having a clean, light, bright and attractive place to eat is also conducive to positive eating habits. Table mats can be used for toddlers and table cloths for older children, with flowers or other table decorations that they have made or arranged.

Most children will eat more comfortably if they have had a period of settling before a meal rather than being rushed from busy activities directly to the meal table. The daily routine can be planned with this in mind, and hand washing can be integrated with some quiet activities such as stories, songs and discussions.

Nutrition activities

There are many activities that can actively promote nutrition with children. These activities should be part of the planned program and not just activities at mealtimes. It is useful to think of nutrition education as being an integral part of the learning experiences that are planned to enhance all areas of child development.

Gardening

Digging in gardens and filling pots with earth before planting seeds or seedlings not only encourages growth and coordination of large muscles but provides an opportunity to think and talk about plants and food. The plants can be observed and differences noticed. Children can observe the differences and similarities between plants and their growth patterns. All of these are very valid science activities.

Being responsible for regular watering also gives the children opportunities for developing independence and personal responsibility. The vegetables can be picked, washed and prepared for eating by the children.

Toddlers cannot cope conceptually with the long time delay needed for growing vegetables in the garden or pots. Children in this age group are best with sprouts and cress grown indoors, where the growth is evident early and where the end result is ready to be eaten within a couple of weeks.

Planting such seeds is a valuable learning experience and toddlers enjoy cutting off the sprouts and making a sandwich (using whole grain bread) for lunch.

Feeding animals

Keeping animals develops a sense of individual responsibility in children. Many children's services keep a small animal such as a guinea pig or rabbit, and children assist with cleaning out the cage and with feeding the pet. Recognising the animal's need for food and the type of food eaten can lead to interesting discussion about food and humans.

Dramatic play

Dramatic play opportunities can be provided that link to food and shopping. Parents are usually very happy to bring in used food packets, though this should always be nutritional food. Cereal and pasta packets, rinsed milk cartons and fruit juice containers can all be used, as well as plastic fruit, vegetables and meat.

Mealtimes can be springboards for wonderful dramatic play. Having a restaurant can involve allocating tasks, which encourages organisation skills, developing menus, decorating tables, having waiters and customers. Taking on another persona is important for the development of empathy, for learning to recognise how another person feels.

Cooking activities

These should involve nutritional food that can be eaten by the children as part of their food for the day. Chocolate crackles and cakes or biscuits with lots of sugar are not appropriate. Cooking experiences are very much linked to maths and science as well as to food. There will be weighing and measuring to be done and the mixing of ingredients together, which will change the texture. Cooking itself will bring about chemical changes due to heat. All this can be observed and discussed by the children.

Cooking can also be a very sociable activity that requires co-operation, sharing and talking together. The eating together brings with it its own personal and group satisfaction.

Stirring, mixing, cutting, chopping, squeezing and grating are all actions that involve large and small muscles as well as muscle coordination. Sensory development is enhanced by the smelling and tasting of food.

Toddlers should also have cooking experiences but these require a little more thought and planning. If preparing foods such as vegetables for soup it is a good idea to microwave the vegetables until soft and let them cool, so that they can be cut by toddlers with plastic knives.

Hygiene, food and cooking activities

All children and staff must wash their hands before commencing cooking activities.

It is recommended that these activities be limited to food that is to be cooked, as there is the danger that germs from the children's hands (not killed by handwashing) will grow in uncooked food. (NHMRC 1997).

It is an enjoyable and nutritionally valuable activity for children to make foods such as fruit salads. The risk of cross infection can be minimised if each child cuts the fruit into an individual bowl marked with his or her name, and this is the fruit they eat at mealtime.

Social and cultural understanding

Food experiences provide almost unlimited opportunities for gaining an understanding of other cultures. The daily menu should reflect the cultural background of the children within the service and be used to introduce new foods to all the children.

An understanding of the children's diverse backgrounds can be extended by stories from other cultures, by pictures, by parents coming to talk to, and cook with, the children. Children can learn how other children live in these cultures, their housing, clothes and language as well as the food they eat.

Special occasions in all cultures are linked to special food. This gives many chances for talking about food, about rituals and the symbolic meanings of significant events.

Language, literature and music

Talking about food is something we all do, and children will need little encouragement. Caregivers just need to make sure there are plenty of opportunities to talk about food.

There are also many stories, rhymes and songs about food, and these are often fun as well as expanding language experiences.

Learning activities

1. Plan a varied and interesting week's menu, containing all the essential nutrients, for each of the age groups mentioned in this chapter.
2. Describe how you might arrange mealtimes with each age group.
3. Suggest some activities that are linked to nutrition and which also encourage:

language development	social development
cognitive development	fine and gross motor skills

4. Find a selection of children's story books about food that you could use with the activities above.
5. Collect a selection of recipes for interesting but nourishing food for a 3-year-old's birthday party.

References

Australian Broadcasting Corporation (1994). *Lots and lots of great music for kids*. EMI, Australia. Compact Disc.

Australian Nutrition Foundation (1982). The healthy diet pyramid.

NHMRC (1992). *Dietary guidelines for Australians*. Canberra, AGPS.

NHMRC (1995). *Dietary guidelines for children and adolescents*. Canberra, AGPS.

NHMRC (1989). *Implementing the dietary guidelines for Australians*. Canberra, AGPS.

NHMRC (1996). *Infant feeding guidelines for health workers*. Canberra, AGPS.

NHMRC (1997). *Staying healthy in child care*. Canberra, AGPS.

Stanton R. (1990). *Food for under fives*. Sydney, Allen and Unwin.

Ure C. Food planning. In: Sebastian P. ed. (1988) *Handle with care: A guide to early childhood administration*. Brisbane, The Jacaranda Press.

Further reading

Bunney C, Williams L. (1996) *Caring for children: Food, nutrition and fun activities*. Sydney, Food and Nutrition Unit, NSW Health.

Karmel A. (1991). *The complete baby and toddler meal planner*. Melbourne, Viking O'Neil Penguin.

NHMRC (1995). *Dietary guidelines for children and adolescents*. Canberra, AGPS.

NHMRC (1996). *Infant feeding guidelines for health workers*. Canberra, AGPS.

NHMRC (1997). *Staying healthy in child care*. Canberra, AGPS.

Nicol D. (1995). *Thought for food*. Canberra, Australian Early Childhood Association.

Books for children

Carle E. (1970). *The very hungry caterpillar*. Harmondsworth, Hamish Hamilton.

Kerr J. (1968). *The tiger who came to tea*. London, Collins.

Tostoy A. (1968). *The great big enormous turnip*. London, Heinemann.

Fox M. (1983). *Possum magic*. Adelaide, Omnibus. (Lots of treat food here.)

CHAPTER 8

Child safety and accident prevention

ALL CHILDREN HAVE a right to be safe and secure in any setting, be it at home, at child care or playing in the park. This chapter is concerned with the physical safety of children; we will discuss child protection in Chapter 9. Child accidents are a serious health problem in most developed countries, including Australia. Accidents cause most deaths and many hospital admissions in children between 1 and 14 years of age.

Keeping children safe is an important part of keeping them healthy. There is a danger of becoming complacent about accidents and seeing them as events that will always happen. But accidents can be prevented. Perhaps if we viewed accidents as a type of disease, then there might be more emphasis placed on the need for prevention.

One of the positive health benefits for children attending child-care centres is that there are less accidents in the centres than there are in homes. Child-care centres should be safe places for children. They have a physical environment that was designed (or modified) for children. The equipment and toys are also designed for children to use. The staff are trained to provide a safe environment and to prevent accidents.

Family day care homes are carefully checked for safety before registration. This ensures that the physical environment is safe. Child safety is also an important part of the orientation program of new caregivers. Ongoing in-service opportunities should aim to reinforce the need for safety measures and safe behaviour.

Caregivers are also advocates for children and have an important role in helping educate children, other child-care staff, parents and the community about child safety. The child-care facility can be a valuable resource to parents who need information about how best to prevent child accidents.

The world can be a dangerous place for children. Let's now look at some aspects of accidents.

Types of accidents

Children are seriously injured and die from many types of accidents, including:

- Motor vehicle accidents
- Drowning (this is the leading cause of death in Australian children under the age of 5 years)
- Pedestrian and bike accidents
- Burns and scalds
- Falls
- Poisoning
- Choking and suffocation
- Electrocution
- Lacerations

Gender and age differences

There is a difference in the rate of fatal accidents between age groups and between boys and girls. There is also a geographical difference.

- Boys of all ages throughout Australia have a much higher accident rate than girls.
- The Northern Territory has by far the highest child death rate in Australia; the lowest is in the Australian Capital Territory.
- The under-6-years-old group have more accidents than others. Children in this age group are developing the physical ability, problem-solving skills and curiosity to get into dangerous places, but are only beginning to develop an understanding of danger. A child of 3 years might see a brightly coloured container of cleaning fluid on a high shelf. His curiosity drives him to want to taste this substance. His problem-solving skills enable him to work out how to get a chair in order to reach the lower shelf, and his physical ability makes it possible for him to climb up onto the higher shelf.

Safety policies in children's services

The rate of childhood accidents means that all children's services must take child safety into account in all parts of their operations. It is the responsibility of the child-care professional:

- to provide a safe environment for children;
- to practise safe behaviour;
- to provide information, resources and assistance to colleagues and parents.

All children's services must aim to prevent accidents from occurring at all. It is very important to develop policies that identify preventive measures and procedures to follow should accidents occur, and which can be practised by *all* staff. Policies for child safety give guidance to all staff and therefore assist them to develop safe practices.

The importance of safety policies is recognised in Government accreditation requirements. Child-care centres will not gain accreditation unless there are written safety policies and the staff are seen to be putting these into practice.

Childhood accidents and child development

Children are in danger of having different types of accidents at different ages and stages of development.

Babies

Babies are at risk of falling from a bed or change table. Even very young babies can wriggle and be in danger of falling. Caregivers need to collect all the equipment and materials needed for nappy changing or bathing and have them ready before getting the baby. Always take the baby with you if you need to get something away from the table. Caregivers must practise safe behaviour, which includes constant supervision.

Babies can slide out of strollers and high chairs and be injured from the fall, or get their neck caught as they slide and strangle themselves. Suitable restraints need to be fitted and used.

Nursery equipment also needs to be well designed so that injuries such as catching legs in the bars of a cot cannot occur.

Crawlers (or creepers)

As a child grows and is able to move, the dangers increase. The child can get into more places, can pick up small objects and put them in her mouth, with the risk of swallowing and inhaling (choking on) these objects.

The crawler can fall down stairs, climb into wading pools and topple into unfenced swimming pools.

Once the crawler has started to stand up and walk around the furniture, she is in danger of pulling heavy articles from shelves and tables onto herself.

Toddlers (12 months to 2½ years of age)

This period is the most dangerous in a child's life. The toddler can move around easily (and often very quickly) but he hasn't got to a stage of knowing about dangerous things. His main aim in life is to explore everything and caregivers need to provide exciting, yet safe, places to explore.

Toddlers enjoy pulling at objects, and this means that dangling tablecloths can be dangerous if there are sharp objects or hot drinks on the table.

Toddlers are also at risk of falling down stairs. Remember that toddlers are able to climb up stairs before they can climb down. Remember, too, that at this age the child is unable to work out heights, as the spatial concepts of height and depth are not yet developed, and this means that they might climb up high and not know it is dangerous.

Water is very interesting to toddlers and is especially dangerous. Drowning is the most common cause of toddler deaths. Swimming and wading pools are the main danger, but children can drown in very shallow water, so laundry buckets, water play troughs, baths and basins are also dangerous.

As toddlers get older they are able to take the tops off bottles of medicines or poisons and open tablet packs. They are also able to climb and problem-solve, so that it is now easy for them to pull out a chair and climb onto a bench to reach high cupboards.

3–5-year-olds

Children between 3 and 5 years of age are becoming more independent and need a safe and secure environment where they can ride bikes, run around, kick balls, climb and try out new activities.

5–12-year-olds

Older children are often out alone and need to be aware of road safety and wear helmets when on bikes. This age group is also at risk of being injured during sporting activities.

Some other developmental issues

Children need to have lots of activities so that they can develop and learn new skills. It is, however, very important to remember that infants, toddlers and young children are unable to tell the difference between safe activities (provided by safety-conscious caregivers) and dangerous activities. Some examples are:

- Pulling toys along on a cord or string is an enjoyable activity for toddlers. However it is important to understand that the toddler is unable to tell the difference between the cord on the pull-along toy and the cord on the electric jug or the hot iron or the dangling tablecloth. Therefore iron and jug cords and dangling tablecloths should be kept totally away from children—or the child away from these unsafe objects.
- Between the ages of 2 and 3, children have begun to be very interested in manipulative equipment (eg. lego, small blocks), which is an important activity and assists with the development of fine movement and co-ordination. At this age the child is unable to tell the difference between all the safe manipulative equipment and the dangerous bottle or packet of pills which he finds in someone's handbag or on a shelf in the bathroom. The child should have lots of safe manipulative equipment with which to play, and unsafe articles should be safely locked away.

Specific dangers to children

Different stages of development have their own dangers. There are specific dangers to children that need special safety measures.

Water

Water plays an important part in a young child's learning but, as we have noted, is also a potential danger to children. Infants, toddlers and young children must always be supervised near water and must never be left alone. This includes the bathroom and laundry as well as other areas of the centre.

Water must also be removed when children have finished playing, eg. emptying of wading pools and water play troughs immediately the activity is over. (Note that some States or Territories may not permit or may strictly limit the use of pools in a child care service. See Chapter 6).

Large wading pools and swimming pools should be fenced, with gates that meet Australian Standards. Many of the pools in child-care centres can be emptied after use, but it should be remembered that empty swimming pools are also a danger because of the risk of falls. Even large puddles and water that has collected in containers after rain are potentially very dangerous to a toddler.

Falls

Falls are the cause of most accidents in child care. Falls can occur by tripping or slipping on flat surfaces as well as from higher places.

Babies

As already noted, infants are in danger of falling from nappy changing tables or beds and should therefore never be left alone. A useful rule for nappy changing time is 'always have one hand on the baby'.

Likewise, older babies are at risk of slipping from high chairs and strollers and therefore need suitable restraints such as baby harnesses. The design of such restraints is also important, as they should be comfortable and allow the child movement. The clasp should also be of a design that babies and toddlers, who are quickly developing manipulative skills, are unable to undo.

Crawlers

Crawling babies need barriers around any stairs. These barriers should be at the top and bottom of the stairs.

The crawling baby who has started to pull herself up will have many falls as she practises her balancing skills. These falls should not harm the baby if the floor surfaces are even and there are no sharp edges on tables or other equipment on which the baby might jab herself.

Toddlers

Once crawlers become toddlers it is important for them to have uncluttered space to walk around so that their gross motor co-ordination develops. It is essential that carers ensure that walking surfaces are even and that there are no obstacles such as toys, blocks and other equipment lying around that the child may trip over. Slipping over on wet surfaces now becomes a concern, so spills need to be wiped up immediately.

Toddlers are great explorers but, as mentioned before, have limited spatial concepts (ideas about how high something is) and no perception of danger. They will excitedly climb equipment that was designed for 4-year-olds and then fall through the spaces on the climbing frame. Providing an exciting and stimulating yet safe place for toddlers to play is of utmost importance.

3–5-year-olds

Young children are often active climbers, and climbing is an important activity. These children need well designed and maintained equipment in order to climb safely. Suitable impact-absorbing material (such as tan or pine bark, or foam mats) should also be placed under all climbing equipment, swings and slides (and trees, too, if this is appropriate).

5–12-year-olds

Older children are becoming increasingly independent and at risk of falls from bikes, play equipment such as monkey bars, as well as skateboards and roller skates. Suitable protective clothing and pads now become important. Mouth guards may be necessary in competitive sports.

Dangerous substances

Dangerous substances can be harmful in many ways—eg. poisons that are swallowed, fumes that are inhaled and corrosive substances that burn the skin when swallowed or touched (your State or Territory office of the Child Accident Prevention Foundation of Australia—Kidsafe—has leaflets covering these poisons).

Children under 5 years of age are more likely to swallow poisons than older children. Younger children are unable to recognise dangerous substances and their natural need to explore and experiment means that they will taste and swallow even the most horrible-tasting substances. Children are also attracted to packets and bottles of pills, which look very much like lollies.

Once children have reached a stage where their motor co-ordination allows them to climb and they are developing problem-solving skills, they will climb to high shelves and other out-of-the-way places where they might find dangerous substances.

All dangerous substances should be kept safely out of reach and locked away from children, using childproof locks. It is very important that the substances be kept away from children at all times.

Play substances such as paint, dyes, crayons and pencils should all be non-toxic so that young children, who need to taste everything (which is a very normal developmental thing to do), will not be harmed.

Heat

Heat from fires, heaters, hot water, and steam can cause fatal injuries to children and cause horrific scarring and disabilities. A child who is badly burnt will have to stay in hospital for a long time and have much pain. Again, it is the younger children (under 5 years of age) who are most at risk.

Children should not be able to come into contact with sources of heat. Here are some safety measures that will reduce the danger of burns and scalds:

- Children should be in the kitchen for cooking and other activities only with adult supervision. There should be barriers in place at all other times to prevent young children having access, and limits about the rules of safety set for older children.
- Ensure that there are no dangling cords, that saucepans have handles turned in and there is, if possible, a stove guard in place.
- All heating appliances should have guards around them.
- The temperature of the water in the hot water service should be controlled so that a child will not get a serious scald from the hot water tap. Child-resistant taps should also be installed in laundries and kitchens.
- Children should always be supervised in the bathroom, which will lessen the risk of taps being turned on.
- Staff should never have hot drinks when young children are around.
- Microwave ovens distribute heat unevenly, so babies' bottles should not be heated this way. Remember to always test the temperature of the milk in the bottle by dripping some onto the inner part of your lower arm. Solid food should be should be stirred to distribute the heat evenly.
- Older children should be given instructions about the dangers of matches and flammable substances.

Sunburn

Heat from the sun is dangerous in both the short and long term. Serious burns can occur when a child is unprotected in the sun, which then raises the likelihood of developing skin cancer later in life. Sunburn should not occur in children's services and all children must be protected.

Children's services should have a sun policy and ensure that children wear a shirt, have sunscreen applied and wear a hat whenever out in the sun. Staff should also wear a hat and protective clothing, both for their own benefit and also in order to provide a role model for the children. Children's services should also have adequate shaded areas where children can play.

Electrical equipment

The home is where most electrical injuries and deaths of children occur. However there must be an awareness of the dangers of electricity in all children's services.

- All electrical equipment should be in good working order with no frayed cords.
- Power points should have suitable covers in place when not in use.

Choking

Children do not have a full set of molars (chewing teeth) until they are around 2 years old. This means that they are in danger of choking on some foods such as nuts and hard pieces of raw carrot and apple, as well as on small, inedible objects left lying around.

- Nuts (apart from peanut and other nut paste/butter) should never be given to children under the age of 5 years.
- Raw apple, carrot and similar food should be grated or given cooked.
- Children should always sit down at meal and snack times.
- Babies should always be nursed when feeding from a bottle and never have the bottle propped.
- Floors should be kept free of small objects.

Suffocation

Babies and toddlers are able to suffocate on plastic sheeting and plastic bags. Caregivers need to ensure that:

- mattress protectors are of a firm waterproof material;
- plastic bags and other soft plastic items are stored away from children; it is a good idea to always tie a knot in plastic bags before storing them;
- there are no dangling cords on curtains or blinds in which children could get their neck caught.

Pedestrian and bike accidents

Before they reach about 8 years of age at least, children are unable to work out the speed of cars and other traffic, nor are children able to tell how quickly the traffic might reach them. This makes it very hard for children to assess when it is safe to cross the road. Children under school age should always be accompanied by an adult.

- Always encourage children to cross roads at a pedestrian crossing or where there are traffic lights. Adults can help by being role models and practising safe behaviour themselves.
- Children should attend road safety classes before riding bikes on roads.
- The simple rule 'No helmet, no bike' should be followed both at home and school.

Lacerations (cuts)

Cuts can occur from sharp objects and from fingers being squashed in doors or other equipment.

- Young children should use round-ended scissors with supervision.
- Sharp objects should be kept away from children.
- Doors should have a seal of rubber or foam around them to prevent jamming.
- Children should not walk around with glass implements in case they fall and the glass breaks.

A safe environment

Other important points that need to be taken into consideration are:

- Making sure that the service's safety policy is being put into practice.
- Having a check-list of all the safety factors in the service that can be regularly assessed.
- Regularly checking to see that equipment is well maintained and repairs carried out when needed. Too often bolts and screws on climbing equipment become loose and stick out, causing lacerations, or the eyes on teddy bears and soft toys loosen and come off and might be inhaled.
- Checking the grounds each morning for unsafe articles that might have been thrown over or through the fence overnight. There have been several cases where used needles and syringes have been found inside the fences of child-care centres.
- Choosing equipment that is designed with safety in mind. This includes all types of equipment, from the design of the fence and gates to the type of utensils used for eating and drinking.
- Taking safety into account when planning all activities, learning experiences and routines.
- Setting up and placing activities in safe places.

- Ensuring that there is constant supervision of all children at all times.

Safe behaviour and safety education

Staff and children should be encouraged to act safely in order to prevent accidents. Seeing staff acting safely is a way of providing safety education for children (for example, wearing hats in the sun).

Children should be constantly supervised. Staff need to position themselves so that they can talk to one child, or a small group of children, while still being able to observe and supervise the rest of the group. Children should never be left alone, and this includes sleeping children.

Staff should make sure that there is adequate planning and preparation of activities and routines. Here are some examples of what can happen if this is not done:

- sending too many children to the bathroom at once, which causes pushing and spilling and slipping over on the floor;
- sitting the toddlers at the table before the meal is ready, so that they become restless with nothing to do and climb onto the table, fall off and knock another child from his chair;
- setting up messy activities (say finger painting) a long way from the bathroom, so that children spill paint onto the floor on their way to the bathroom and someone slips on the paint;
- not having enough equipment for children; one bucket and spade in the sandpit with three toddlers will quickly lead to the child with the bucket and spade hitting the others as they try to take the implements from him.

Limits should be set for children. These limits, of course, depend on the age of the child.

- Taking turns—one person on the slide at a time is fine for 3-year-olds and over, but you will need to distract the younger children with other activities until it is their turn.
- Give positive directions, with an explanation; eg. to a running child: 'Walk inside, Mary. You might fall when you run'. Otherwise you'll find yourself always saying 'don't'.
- Keep children a safe distance from the swings (swings should ideally be places away from main areas and have a low barrier around them).
- Have rules for older children about wearing of safety equipment such as bike helmets and mouth guards.

Community health resources

Staff in children's services play an important role in parent education. Leaflets and brochures on child safety and accident prevention should be available and displayed for parents to see. This means that staff need to be aware of useful child safety resources that are available from other organisations. Many such resources are available from the Child Accident Prevention Foundation of Australia (Kidsafe), which has an office in all capital cities.

In-service programs are also important as they allow staff to keep up to date with new information and practices. Organisations such as the Road Safety Authority have also developed safety kits for children.

Excursions and travelling with children

Excursions provide a range of experiences for children. There is the opportunity to see new places, events and people. Taking a group of children on an excursion requires careful preparation. There are also legal requirements that must be taken into account.

Parent permission

It is an essential legal requirement that parents give written permission for their child to leave the centre or other children's service at any time.

This permission may be ongoing, eg. for a child to be taken to preschool daily, but for one-off occasions such as a special excursion a special form needs to be signed. The parents should be given plenty of notice about:

- when and why the excursion is happening;
- where you are going;
- how you are travelling;
- which staff and adults are going to travel with the children;
- any special clothes the child might need to wear, eg. shoes, hats, rain coats;
- any special items the child may need to bring, eg. cups, towel;
- any cost involved.

It may also be necessary to have permission forms and information about the excursion translated into the parents' language. Many parents come from a non-English speaking background.

Regulations relating to staff/child ratios

Each State and Territory has regulations regarding staff/child ratios when chidren are outside the child-care centre. The following is a general guideline:

- one adult for every two children under 3 years of age;
- one adult for every three children 3–5 years old;
- one adult for every eight children aged 6 years and over;
- for groups of more than 15 children, one extra person in charge should be available.

Extra staff will be needed if the excursion is to be to a place that has environmental or traffic dangers, such as being near water or having to cross a busy road.

Centre communication

The following information about the excursion must always be left at the child-care centre (or other children's service):

- a copy of your proposed route of travel and the destination;
- contact phone numbers or a mobile phone number if possible;
- a copy of your time schedule, which includes destination arrival and departure times as well as your estimated time of arrival back at the centre;
- a copy of the names of children and adults on the excursion.

Constant supervision

The need for constant supervision has been mentioned before and the importance of this is emphasised again, not only while travelling but also while at your destination. Remember, too, that children may need to use public toilet facilities and will need adult supervision at this time.

Planning

Planning ahead helps to anticipate any particular problems that might occur. Planning also helps identify if there will be any times when the children might be kept waiting and become restless, so you can arrange to have appropriate activities such as songs.

It is also a good idea to check the details of your planned excursion the day before in case of transport strikes, road closures or other unforeseen events.

Preparing the children for the excursion will include setting safety limits that are appropriate to each age group.

Untoward incidents

There are reporting procedures that need to be followed if an incident or accident happens. Each child-care setting has its own incident forms and procedures for reporting and these must be strictly followed, as this is a legal requirement.

Safe collection and return of children

It is often useful to discuss the outing with other staff and identify how you will collect, transport and return the children. Some of the questions you need to address are:

- Will all the children leave from the children's service or might some parents bring their children to the excursion venue?
- Are all children going back to the children's service, or will some parents collect children from the excursion venue before you return?

A list of the names of all the children going on the excursion is essential and it is important on the day to check that all these children are in attendance and have come on the excursion with you. It is also essential that you check the names of these children before and after returning from the excursion.

It is a good idea to have a written plan with a check-list of all the important points you need to remember on the day. These may include items you need to take such as:

- food for children and staff;
- water and cups;
- first aid kit;
- ground sheet or blanket;
- strollers for younger children;
- extra nappies and spare pairs of pants;
- damp tissues for wiping hands and faces;
- extra sunscreen;
- sun-hats for all children;
- mobile phone, phone cards or cash for public phones.

Types of transport

The type of transport used will depend on:

- the age of the children;
- distance between the children's service and where the outing is being held;
- availability of parents to help;

- access to public transport;
- available transport at children's service, such as mini-bus;
- cost;
- number of children and adults going on excursion.

Some types of transport might be:

- walking, if the venue is not far away;
- parents' cars (it is essential that these cars are registered and that drivers have a current driving licence);
- mini-bus (and that the driver has the correct driving licence for that type of vehicle and that it is equipped with suitable restraints for the age/weight of each child);
- hired transport such as a bus;
- public transport such as bus, tram or train.

Safety equipment

Road accidents are one of the greatest causes of death and injury among children. These accidents include deaths when children are passengers in a car and when pedestrians.

Accidents can also happen when children are transported in prams or strollers, and falls and strangulation can occur because correct restraints are not used. It is absolutely essential that the correct restraints are used for each child.

- Prams and strollers need correctly fitted and comfortable restraints that are used at ALL times.
- Restraints in cars must be Australian Standards approved and be correctly installed in the rear seat.
- Restraints in cars must be appropriate to the weight and stage of development of the child, eg. baby capsules, car seats, booster seats and the correct safety harness for 3–11 year olds who are using the rear seat belts (there are a range of these harnesses to suit the age and weight of children).

Walking with children

It is important that children less than 4–5 years of age hold an adult's hand when crossing roads or in busy or crowded areas. Older children might hold each other's hands and cross roads under the supervision of adults. All children should have road safety education and this should start as soon as the child can walk, even if they are still in strollers.

Excursion backpack

This is a backpack set up especially for outings or excursions where you will be walking. The backpack could contain items such as a first aid kit, mobile phone, emergency phone numbers, spare items of clothing, sunscreen and tissues.

Safety of children during travel

Specific safety measures are needed for each type of transport that might be used to transport children on an excursion.

Cars

Child-care staff need to ensure that all children are sitting comfortably in the appropriate restraints and that these restraints are correctly fastened. A check should be made to ensure that no harness straps are rubbing parts of the child's body. Care needs to be taken on hot days that the seat covering or the metal on buckles is not too hot.

Where possible, it is helpful to have an adult other than the driver in the car. This extra person can then chat to the children about what is happening outside the car, such as places they are passing, trucks and buses on the road.

Children can become restless sitting in a car, so plan songs to sing or have tapes to play, and have books or other appropriate activities to entertain them.

Mini-bus

This form of transport should be fitted with appropriate child restraints and staff need to ensure that children are correctly and comfortably sitting in these restraints before starting the bus. Extra staff or adults should sit with the children to chat with them and supervise safety.

Public transport

It is difficult travelling on public transport with babies and toddlers unless there is one adult per child.

Older children enjoy this form of transport (many families' main form of transport is the car, so it is a new experience for some children to travel on public transport). Children need to be well prepared for travel on public transport and staff need to have checked timetables well in advance so that there are no groups of restless children waiting at bus stops or train stations. It is often a good idea to provide some dramatic play activities relating to travel prior to the excursion and to chat with the children about the limits set for the excursion.

Again, it is a legal requirement that there are sufficient adults present on these excursions. It is very important that all children are constantly supervised during travel and while on the excursion.

Dangerous situations

There are many reasons why situations in child care can become dangerous. (An overview of first aid principles is given following these case studies.)

CASE STUDY 1: CHILDREN

James is just over 2½ years old and is the very proud owner of some new boots. He has also just learned how to jump for long periods on the jumping board and spends much of his time outdoors doing this.

Anna is 11 months old and is able to pull herself up and walk around furniture and other sturdy equipment. She crawls over to the jumping board and places her hands on the board just as James does an especially large bounce. The staff are alerted by Anna's scream and she is found to have lacerated and bleeding fingers.

This example describes two children who are behaving in exactly the right way for children of their ages, yet this normal behaviour causes a dangerous situation. James is jumping and does not realise that he may land on Anna's fingers. Anna is completely unaware of the danger.

Anna is screaming and her fingers are bleeding. You would immediately pick Anna up or sit with her on your lap, checking at the same time that James is unharmed. Soothing Anna and checking her fingers would be the first thing to do. It is also a good idea to keep a pair of disposable plastic gloves in your pocket, which you should put on before touching Anna's bleeding fingers.

CASE STUDY 2: STAFF

Despina, who is 15 months old, has just started walking and is becoming increasingly mobile, though she still stumbles and trips on objects and uneven surfaces. She wanders into the 3–5-year-olds' area through a gate left open when the children went indoors for morning tea. There is an unattended wading pool in this area. Despina leans over the wading pool to pick up a leaf and is found with her head down in the water.

In this case study, Despina is at a stage where she is an active explorer yet still a little unsteady on her feet. Staff have left a gate open as well as leaving a potentially dangerous item unattended, ie. the wading pool. Nor, it seems, was there any supervision of Despina at this time.

Despina may be seriously injured—she could be unconscious, she could have hurt limbs or other parts of her body when tripping over. Your initial response would be to remove her from danger (the water) and to then assess the situation.

CASE STUDY 3: EQUIPMENT

Ngyen, who is just over 4 years of age, is climbing on the highest part of the climbing frame. He enjoys the physical challenge of the climbing. The climbing frame has not been well maintained and is also wet due to recent rain.

Ngyen slips from the top and cuts his arm badly on a bolt that is poking out. He also lands on the ground, where the impact-absorbing material has worn thin. Staff rush over to him and find him holding his leg and sobbing that it hurts, while bleeding freely from his arm.

There are many causes for this accident, but the main reasons are lack of maintenance of the climbing frame and not enough impact-absorbing material on the ground. The rain has also caused the climbing frame to become slippery.

Ngyen's conscious state is evident from his sobbing, but before you assess Ngyen you need to quickly check that there is no-one else up the climbing frame who could fall on you both.

CASE STUDY 4: CENTRE ROUTINE

It is afternoon tea time and the staff bring out some nutritious raw vegetables and dips. All the children are outdoors; they take their food and run off to play while eating. Antonio is 16 months old and takes a piece of raw carrot. He also wanders off and starts pushing a pram around, when he suddenly starts coughing violently and falls to the ground.

It is essential that the centre routine takes safety measures into account. All children should sit down to eat, not be given food while they are wandering around. Children under 2 years should also not be given raw carrot to eat, or other hard foods on which there is any danger of choking.

Antonio may be a real emergency if the carrot is blocking his airway, and you need to quickly assess the situation.

CASE STUDY 5: SETTING UP ACTIVITIES

A finger-painting activity using shaving cream has been set up for a group of 2–3-year-olds. It has been set up some way from the bathroom and there are no towels to wipe hands on. Phillipa drips some of the shaving cream on the way to the bathroom and Tony, who is walking past, slips and falls backwards to the floor, hitting his head hard. He does not respond when staff reach him.

Safety is an important consideration when setting up activities. A messy activity (and messy activities are valuable for young children) should be placed near a bathroom, or towels should be available for each child so that there is no (or minimum) risk of spilling and slipping.

Tony may have serious injuries, which need to be immediately assessed

(ANTA 1997).

Other children

In all these situations it is important that staff remain calm and give reassurance and comfort to the injured child. Other children may also be distressed, so they will also need reassurance and another staff member should take them to another activity in an area away from the injured child.

Principles of first aid

It is not within the scope of this book to give detailed descriptions of first aid. All trained staff in child care will have a Senior First Aid Certificate. The best text is the most recent handbook (or CD Rom) from St John's Ambulance, *Australian first aid*.

There are, however, some assessment procedures that must be carried out in the case of an emergency:

1. Check for danger to see that no other children or staff are in danger of being hurt or that the injured child will not be further hurt.
2. Check the injured child's response, which is an assessment of their conscious state. A lack of response indicates the seriousness of the situation and the following should be immediately checked:

- that the airway is clear;
- that the child is breathing;
- that there is a pulse (circulation).

3. You will also need to examine the whole body for:
   - bleeding;
   - fractures;
   - other serious injuries.

Further action

In all cases you need to assess the situation very quickly and respond to the emergency. You may be the first person to reach the child, but always alert another staff member in a dangerous situation. Your initial assessment of the injured child is most important because you will need to decide if:

- the child is unconscious and needs to be placed on their left side;
- you need to commence mouth-to-mouth or cardiopulmonary resuscitation;
- the injury is so serious that an ambulance needs to be called immediately;
- the injuries are serious enough for the child to need immediate medical attention;
- the injuries are minor but the parents need to be called to take the child home;
- the injuries are minor and the child can be treated in the centre.

A list of emergency numbers should be placed near the phone, in a position where it is easily seen.

Calling an ambulance

Ambulances are called in emergency situations. It is important that the ambulance arrives as soon as possible.

All staff should know the procedure regarding calling 000, which is used in an emergency for fire, police and ambulance. You should:

- ask the operator for the service you need;
- wait to be connected.

When speaking to the ambulance service you should:

- state the exact location of the accident, giving the address and position very clearly;
- state the type of injury;

- ensure that the ambulance, both vehicle and officers, have easy access to the injured child. You may need to take the other children to another part of the centre in order to lessen their distress and to keep the access area clear.

Emergency evacuation procedures

It may be necessary to evacuate the centre in the case of fire or a bomb threat. Fire and evacuation drills are an important safety measure in any children's service and you should become familiar with these procedures.

Legal requirements

Minor accidents

All untoward incidents and accidents (no matter how small) must be reported to a senior staff member and entered in the Accident Book (your service might have another name for this book).

A verbal report of the accident or incident must be given to the parent when they collect their child that day.

Serious accidents

On enrolment of their child in the centre, each parent or guardian will sign a form authorising the child-care centre staff to seek medical attention or call an ambulance in the case of an emergency.

Parents must always be IMMEDIATELY notified in an emergency situation. A list of emergency contact numbers for parents should be listed in the children's records

All action taken in an emergency situation must be accurately documented in writing. This is a legal requirement and the written report may be used as evidence in a court of law.

Accident prevention and the community

Three main points have been identified in relation to the community and child accident prevention (Pearn 1982). These are:

- Education
- Design
- Legislation.

Education

It is essential that child-care professionals and parents are aware of the need for safety when working and living with children. The whole community also needs to be educated as to the seriousness of child accidents. The more people who think that child safety is an important health issue, the better the chance of preventing accidents occurring.

Design

Design plays a major part in accident prevention and safety. This includes equipment such as nursery furniture, child restraints, toys and clothes that are specifically designed for children. The design of general domestic equipment such as electrical appliances and household furniture is also an important factor in child safety. Australian Standards now apply to many household appliances, children's furniture and structures such as home buildings and swimming pool fences.

Well designed equipment is becoming more easily available. In many capital cities there is a Kidsafe house where information about safe equipment can be obtained. The building industry has a Kidsafe Home project that is committed to designing homes for families with young children. Some of the safety features they have looked at are safe power points, controlled hot water thermostats to prevent scalding, vertical rails on verandahs to prevent climbing, and safe windows to prevent falls.

Legislation

Legislation is often enacted when there have been many accidents from a specific cause. An example is the law on child restraints in cars. (It is worth noting that restraints were required for adults some years before they were required for children.)

There are laws relating to the wearing of bicycle helmets in most parts of Australia. Isolation fencing for swimming pools is also a legal requirement by State law or local council regulation in most parts of Australia.

Various Consumer Affairs Acts and the Trade Practices Act means that dangerous items can be withdrawn from sale and banned. This tends to happen after a child has been killed or badly injured by such a product.

Advocacy

Children have legal rights within our society but are usually unable to voice their needs. Child-care professionals and other adults can be advocates for the rights of children. This is an important part of ensuring a safe environment where children can flourish without being harmed.

Learning activities

1. Contact your nearest Kidsafe Centre and collect some publications.
2. Design an indoor and outdoor safety check-list for a family day-care home.

References

Australian Institute of Health and Welfare. (1998). *Australia's health 1998: The sixth biennial health report of the Australian Institute of Health and Welfare*. Canberra, AIHW.

Australian National Training Authority (1997). CHC019: *Accident prevention and child protection, Melbourne,* ACTRAC Products Ltd.

National Child Care Accreditation Council (1993). *Putting children first. Quality improvement and accreditation system handbook*. Sydney, NCAC.

Pearn J. (1982). *The prevention of childhood accidents: Design, education and legislation*. Glebe, Australasian Medical Publishing Company.

St John Ambulance Australia. (1999). *First aid for children fast*. Sydney, Dorling Kindersley.

Further reading

Publications from Child Accident Prevention Foundation of Australia (Kidsafe) in all capital cities and the Hunter Region, NSW.

CHAPTER 9

Child protection

PROTECTING CHILDREN FROM harm is one of the basic principles of child care in all settings. Parents, child-care and health professionals, as well as others in the community, all work towards keeping children safe.

As has been discussed in previous chapters, the threat to children's physical, social and emotional wellbeing comes from various sources. There is the harm that can happen *in utero*, the harm from infection, poor nutrition and from accidents. There is also the harm that can come from those who are in positions of trust in a child's life, people who are loved and who are responsible for caring for the child. This is the harm of child abuse.

Child abuse is a very serious and distressing topic and raises issues of social health, the rights of children and the needs of families. It is very easy, and understandable, to become emotional when working with a child who has been, or who is being, abused. It may help to look at child abuse as a social illness. As with any other illness, the emphasis is on prevention.

Child-care staff spend more time with children than anyone else apart from the parents, thus they are in a very special position to recognise and help prevent child abuse.

Historical aspects

In the past, children have often been used and abused in ways that would not now be tolerated in our society. Some societies practised female infanticide or physically painful customs such as binding girls' feet. Young children were often sent to work in factories and in other very unsafe situations. Child labour still happens in some countries of the world.

The practice of female circumcision (where the clitoris is removed) is a cultural ritual in some African communities. Recently there have been international protests about this practice, which is not only cruel and dangerous, but inhibits sexual pleasure when the child has grown to womanhood. Male circumcision, which involves removing penile foreskin, is seen as a cultural ritual and a health practice. Though it may be an initially painful procedure unless done soon after birth, it is seldom life-threatening and does not prevent sexual enjoyment for a man. Female circumcision is an issue where the need to object to real cruelty outweighs the acceptance of the rituals of other cultures.

Children were often severely punished in the past. In the domestic situation it was accepted that parents, usually fathers, had a right to discipline children as they saw fit. This discipline was often very harsh and involved beating the child in a way that would nowadays be seen as physical abuse. 'Spare the rod and spoil the child' was a Biblical injunction that parents took seriously as part of child-rearing practices.

Children whose parents had died or who were otherwise unable to care for them were often placed in large institutions. The staff at these institutions were frequently untrained and unsuited to child care. The full extent of the abuse carried out in these institutions is still becoming public. The abused children often had no one to confide in and hid the abuse, both physical and sexual, as a shameful secret. This has caused great life-long emotional harm.

The practice of taking Aboriginal children from their parents persisted into the 1970s and many adults are still feeling the very real pain caused by being deprived of culture and family.

The current situation

It would be comforting to think that cruelty to children was a thing of the past. Young children in Australia may not be sent out to work, as happens in many developing countries; the days when many children were sent to live in large institutions are over. Yet there are still many children who are being abused and need protection.

We now formally recognise the rights of the child as declared by the United Nations in the 1989 Convention on the Rights of the Child. We also recognise that childhood is a very special time and that child-care professionals have an ethical responsibility to ensure the child is safe and protected from harm. All children have a right to feel safe and secure and this, of course, is intrinsic to the aims of all child care.

In a landmark article in the *Journal of the American Medical Association* in 1962, Kempe et al. described 'the battered child syndrome'. Their description of child abuse as a 'syndrome' really drew the attention of health professionals and the general public to what was happening to children.

In Australia, Birrel (1968) described the 'maltreatment syndrome' in children by looking at the injuries of children in hospital.

Many years later, child abuse is still with us and the statistics show that the number of reports of suspected child abuse is rising quite dramatically.

Child abuse statistics

In 1997 Briggs and Hawkins reported that, in the 12 months ending 30 June 1994, 74,436 reports of child abuse and neglect were made to the authorities. This was a 26% increase over the previous year. Just under half of all the reports investigated were found to be cases of child abuse.

More recent figures show that the numbers of notifications continue to rise in most States and Territories. There were 98,568 notifications of suspected child abuse at a national level in 1997–98. Some 26,024 of these cases were confirmed. The difference between the number of notifications and confirmations may be because the community is more aware of the need for child protection and so report suspected cases of abuse more often (AIHW 1999).

What is child abuse?

The term 'child abuse' is very broad. There are sometimes grey areas, where it is hard to decide what constitutes child abuse.

- Is the child whose parents believe a quick smack is part of child rearing an abused child? Parents who do not believe in smacking at any time may think such a child is abused.
- What about the child who gets sunburnt in a child-care setting? Child-care staff should all know how to prevent sunburn and the importance of doing so. It this a case of child neglect on the part of the staff?
- What about the father who yells at his child in the shopping centre? Many people would think that yelling constitutes emotional abuse.

- And what about the mother who leaves her 6-months-old baby on the couch while she answers the doorbell? The baby falls from the couch and fractures his skull. Is this a case of child abuse through neglect?
- A family has certain beliefs about diet and their child is found to be ill and deficient in certain essential nutrients. Is this child abuse?

General definitions of abuse

The following definitions serve as guidelines only to the several categories of abuse. Very often children are abused in more than one way. Sexual abuse includes physical and emotional abuse of the child. The neglected child also suffers emotional and physical abuse through not having emotional and physical needs met.

Physical abuse is a non-accidental (or intentional) injury that occurs as a result of actions, or of failure to act, on the part of parents or guardians/caregivers.

Sexual abuse is where a dependent and developmentally immature child or adolescent is involved in sexual activities that they do not understand and cannot give informed consent to. Sexual abuse as incest also breaks the social rules of our culture concerning what should happen within a family (Oates & Donnelly 1989).

Child neglect is where the needs of children are not met. These can be physical, social, emotional and general developmental needs. Physical neglect is often noticed first, as the child may not have enough—or the wrong—food to eat, be inadequately or inappropriately dressed, or show a general lack of care.

Emotional abuse is where the child is not emotionally supported, valued or respected. He/she may often be shouted at in an abusive way. The child may also be treated in a way that is inappropriate for his/her stage of development. Toddlers may be expected to behave in a rational way and be severely chastised for not sharing, for taking toys from others. Emotional abuse often goes with child neglect, when parents or other caregivers show anger at having to give attention to the child.

Recognising child abuse

There are some signs and symptoms that almost certainly indicate child abuse, though it is often difficult to get a clear picture of what is happening. There may be many signs which, when grouped together, lead caregivers to suspect child abuse. The child should be observed carefully and observations recorded, taking regard of confidentiality.

Recorded observations may be needed by statutory authorities or courts in order to establish that child abuse has occurred. Caregivers do not have the responsibility of diagnosing child abuse but must be alert to the need for child protection.

Physical abuse

There are many injuries that would be difficult to sustain in the usual energetic activities of a child's day. These are injuries that almost certainly are non-accidental and have been inflicted by another person. Injuries such as:

- Cigarette burns, burns from irons or other hot objects that have a distinctive shape.
- Scalds that show that a child has been plunged into hot water, such as scalds to the feet or buttocks.
- Marks on the body that show a child has been hit with a stick, rope, belt, electrical cord or hard object.

There are other injuries that could be caused accidentally, but which should be of concern to caregivers.

- *Black eye/s*: The eye sockets of young children protrude, and it is unlikely that a black eye is the result of a child running into a door. Falling on the sharp edge of a coffee table or other piece of furniture can happen.
- *Bruising*: This is often a difficult sign to interpret. A child may show signs of physical injury such as bruising, but in the usual daily activities there are bumps and falls that can cause bruises to happen. Bruising on the face, back, the buttocks and backs of thighs should be carefully noted and reported to a senior staff member, as should repeated injuries.

  Some children have darker coloured skin around the base of their spine. This is called a Mongolian blue spot and is natural and well documented. This coloured skin is very common in non-Caucasian children and has often been mistaken for bruising. Not a few Asian parents have been suspected of child abuse because child-care and teaching staff have not known about this phenomenon.

There are other injuries for which medical attention is sought and which need to be carefully assessed by health and welfare professionals in order to ascertain whether abuse has occurred.

- Fractures in babies who are not yet mobile always raise the question of non-accidental injury. Very young babies cannot injure themselves. They can fall, however, if left on change tables or other items of furniture. This then raises the question of neglect.

- A brain haemorrhage in a young baby is of grave concern, as this injury can occur when a baby is shaken. Medical staff would always ascertain if there is any brain disease or history of birth trauma present. In the absence of any other cause of the haemorrhage, child abuse would certainly be probable.

Sexual abuse

- Sexual abuse must be seriously considered if a child has genital injuries or bleeding from vagina or anus. The child certainly needs medical attention.
- The child may also show advanced sexual knowledge for their age, be aggressive or withdrawn, and have sleep disturbances.
- There may be other signs that show an inappropriate interest or concern about genitalia and sexuality. These signs are over and beyond the natural interest in all parts of the body that is shown by young children.

Child neglect

- A baby or child who seems to be thin and underweight for age may be suffering from physical neglect. There could be a medical explanation for this condition, which would be discussed and recorded on enrolment.
- Other signs of physical neglect could be unwashed clothes, body and hair, and general poor health.
- A neglected child shows the results of a general lack of care in all areas of development. His verbal and socialisation skills may be poor. He may frequently be tired, as his bedtimes are erratic.
- The child may have many accidents at home.

Behaviour of parent and child

The behaviour of both child and parents can also be an indicator of child abuse.

- Parents' interaction with children may be seriously inconsistent. They may be over-strict or ignore their child.
- Parents may verbally abuse children, threaten and use physical punishment.
- Parents may try to explain away injuries their child has received or give no explanation at all.

- A child may show extremes of passivity (quietness and non-involvement) and be wary when approached by other children and staff. These behaviours are of concern when they are ongoing rather than happening only occasionally. All children (and adults too) will have days when they feel miserable and wish to sit quietly and not join in activities with others.
- Alternatively, an older child may demonstrate extremes of attention-seeking behaviour that is not appropriate for her age.
- Children may be destructive and use aggression to get what they want.

Child abuse by child-care staff

In most cases of child abuse, children are abused by parents or persons who are very close to the family. There have also been cases of staff abusing children in their care. Too often this abuse has been carried out by persons who were well known by the child and in positions of authority and trust.

The breaking of this trust has very understandably made many parents and children worried and anxious about other persons, such as teachers and caregivers, who are in frequent and close contact with children. Male teachers and caregivers are perhaps the most vulnerable to suspicion.

Caregivers can develop and regain this trust by providing a warm and safe environment where physical contact with the child is non-threatening and appropriate for the child's age and stage of development.

Preventing child abuse

Working in a child-care setting means that caregivers are sometimes the first people many parents see in the morning after a sleepless night with a crying baby or a restless toddler. The caregiver is also often the last adult a single parent may speak to after a tiring day at work and before an even more tiring evening of preparing the evening meal and other household tasks. None of this leaves much time for the enjoyable aspects of child rearing such as reading a story or just sitting and having a cuddle.

Staff within a child-care setting may be the first people to recognise that all is not well with a child or within a family. Child abuse happens in all sorts of families—educated, well-off parents may abuse and neglect a child as well as those parents who are struggling to make ends meet.

It is important to listen to parents. It is also important to be aware of body language as well as what the parents are indicating verbally. A parent may be desperately sending out signals for help before they get to the stage of abusing their child. A sympathetic person who shows understanding can help these parents and could prevent the abuse from occurring.

It may be necessary to talk with a more senior staff member who can arrange for the parents to be referred to a community agency for help. Parents who are at risk of abusing their children are often unable to cope with the demands of children. They may suffer from poor self-esteem and feel inadequate about child rearing. Linking up with a community agency may give the support needed so that abuse is prevented.

Adults need to listen to children and respect what a child has told them. One of the real tragedies about abuse (especially sexual abuse) is that children have not been believed when they tried to tell an adult about the abuse. Also, children may not know that such behaviour is not 'normal', or they may be intimidated or threatened by the abuser to keep quiet. Other children have felt so strongly that they would not be believed that they have not attempted to tell an adult. Children need to know that there is a trusting and trusted adult to whom they can go for help, and you may be that person.

Community health and other resources

There are many resources and much information available for families, children and children's services staff. Some places to go are Community Health Centres, Child Protection Agencies, parents' groups and the National Association for Prevention of Child Abuse and Neglect. The Institute of Family Studies provides information for professionals through the National Child Protection Clearinghouse.

Reporting suspected child abuse

This is a very important, albeit sometimes difficult, responsibility for child-care professionals. It is not the role of the child-care professional to prove that a child has been abused. That is the responsibility of health and social workers working within the child-protection agency. The responsibility of the child-care professional is:

- to know the children in his/her care and their families;

- to carefully and sensitively observe the children and their interaction with parents;
- to note and record when child abuse is suspected;
- to keep the records in a safe place;
- to discuss the concerns with a senior staff member;
- to seek advice from a child protection agency if unsure about whether a report should be made;
- to report the suspicions of abuse to the relevant child-protection authority.

One of the important ethical issues is that it is absolutely essential that your knowledge of children and their parents is kept strictly confidential. You must report any concerns you have to a senior staff member or to the Director, but this must be done in private and in the strictest confidence.

Observations must be exact and there needs to be a written record. These observations will be taken very seriously by the child-protection agency personnel, who will use them as evidence when deciding whether the child has been, or is being, abused. These observations might also need to be used in a court of law.

In some child-care settings it is the responsibility of a senior staff member to report any case of suspected child abuse. There have been situations where a senior staff member has been unwilling to report the suspicions in a particular case. A junior staff member who is concerned, on good evidence, for the welfare of the child should then be the person who reports the case of suspected child abuse to the authorities.

Each State and Territory has its own regulations regarding the reporting of child abuse. Each child-care setting should have a copy of these regulations. All staff should have an understanding of the regulations. Reporting is mandatory in all States and Territories except Western Australia.

Policies relating to child protection

Policies relating to the prevention, recognition and reporting of suspected child abuse are needed in children's services and must follow the State or Territory regulations. These policies should be shared with all parents when the child is first enrolled in the child-care setting. New and relief staff must be totally familiar with the policies.

The procedures for identifying, recording and reporting suspected child abuse should be clearly set out. There should be clear policy guidelines relating to staff and the prevention of child abuse.

- Staff credentials and references should be checked before commencing employment.
- Checks should be made to ensure that potential staff do not have convictions for child abuse.
- Attendance at pre- and in-service courses on child abuse should be a regular part of staff training.
- The child-care setting should set out practice guidelines that ensure that children are not alone with only one staff member. Another staff member should always be present or within sight.
- Ensure that students and volunteers are always supervised.
- Family day caregivers should have regular visits from service co-ordinators.
- The design of the child-care setting and the setting up of the environment should facilitate observations of both children and staff.

Physical contact with children

Children need to have a safe and secure environment in which to grow and fully develop emotionally, socially and in all other developmental areas. This means that staff must be sensitive to the changing ages and stages of child development.

- Babies need the comfort and security of being held in a caregiver's arms and gently rocked and stroked. They also need physical care such as being bathed, having nappies changed and being fed.
- Toddlers are becoming much more independent, yet still need support in their physical care. Toddlers will wish to try things such as dressing and going to the toilet themselves. A sensitive caregiver encourages this and gently offers assistance but does not take over the activity from the child. A toddler also needs emotional reassurance and physical comfort from caregivers.
- Young children of 3–5 years of age still need physical comfort and reassurance. They can also start to recognise the difference between the reassurance of physical comfort and inappropriate physical contact.
- As children grow older, the need for privacy gets stronger. This need for privacy must be respected. Remember that many girls have their first menstrual period before 12 years of age, and this is a very private matter. Very frequently, verbal comfort replaces the

child's need for physical comfort with people outside the child's family.

Guidelines for safe practices

Many children's services do not as yet have formal policies relating to physical contact with children. It is difficult to write such a policy for a range of children's ages. What is appropriate physical contact with a baby, such as cuddling, is totally inappropriate for 12-year-olds. Yet we still want to provide for a child's emotional needs at all stages of their development.

Many staff are apprehensive about physical contact with children or how this physical contact might be interpreted. Men are being encouraged to become part of the child-care profession and this is part of equal opportunity practice. Many male students, however, admit to having feelings of uncertainty about how their role in child care is perceived, especially with young children.

- Babies and toddlers need to be washed, bathed and have nappies changed. These routines involve cleaning the genital area. This should be done gently, as you would to any other part of the child's body.
- Activities should be appropriate. It is fun to play 'Round and round the garden . . .' with babies and toddlers and tickle gently under the arm. This sort of game and tickle becomes inappropriate as children get older and pre-adolescent.
- It is essential to remember and respect the growing child's need for privacy and to recognise that their body is their own, and special to them. At the same time there is a need to provide a caring and secure environment. Trusted adults who are respectful of the child's needs are an important part of this environment.
- Many primary schools (and some pre-schools) are now providing Protective Behaviours Programs relating to child sexual abuse. These programs aim to give the child the confidence and ability to recognise when an adult's touch is not OK and how to say NO!
- Caregivers need to be aware of cultural practices that might make it taboo for a male outside of a family to care for a female child, no matter how young the child. There needs to be sensitive discussion with parents from non-Anglo-Australian backgrounds in order to ascertain what are acceptable cultural practices for physical contact with children.

(ANTA1997)

Some situations for concern

CASE STUDY 1

Alex is 2½ years old. He has been attending a long-day care centre part-time for 3 months. He lives with his mother, father and 3-month-old sister in a small flat not far from the child-care centre. Neither parent is in full-time paid work, though the father does have some casual work for a few days each month.

The flats where Alex lives are on a busy road and there is no fenced area for children to play. Many of the other residents are retired and are often at home all day. Some of the other residents have complained to the owners of the flats about the noise Alex and his sister make. It was because of these complaints that Alex's mother called into the child-care centre to ask if he could go there full-time. At that time there were no full-time places available but arrangements were made for Alex to attend the centre for three half-days a week. His parents are eligible for Child Care Benefit for this amount of time.

Staff have noticed that Alex tends to be withdrawn and not even involve himself in parallel play in places such as the sandpit. He becomes very upset if another child approaches him, and hits out and screams. He seems quite happy when left alone with some toys and enjoys his meal and snack times if not placed too near other children.

Staff are concerned about Alex's physical growth. He is very thin and seems much shorter than other children his age. He has not attended a Community Health Centre since he was a small baby and his immunisation is incomplete.

Staff are also concerned about some dark bruises on the back of his body. Discussions with his father (who usually brings and picks up Alex) is that Alex is very clumsy and keeps banging into the furniture. This has not been observed at the centre. The father seems disinclined to discuss the matter further.

It is noted that the father is very curt with Alex and never says goodbye to him. One day Alex did a painting and the staff were pleased to see him enjoy doing this. His father, however, refused to take it home, saying he didn't want such junk cluttering up the flat.

Learning activities I

1. What are the physical and behavioural signs that might indicate that Alex is being abused?
2. What are the specific stresses on Alex's family?
3. Children who have been abused are sometimes enrolled in a child-care centre where the staff can help both the child and the parent/s. How could this happen in Alex's situation?

There are more questions after the next case study.

CASE STUDY 2

Erica is almost 5 years of age and attends family day care full-time. She has been in child care since she was 6 weeks old and attended several child-care centres before coming to family day care 6 months ago. She attends a private pre-school each morning.

Erica lives with her parents and a 12-year-old brother. Her parents both have senior managerial positions in large organisations and work long hours. They are often very late picking up Erica, and the caregiver has discussed this with them several times.

There are 3 other children in family day care with Erica: a baby of 4 months and twin boys who are 2 years old. Erica is an articulate child with a bright personality but the caregiver is concerned about her interaction with the other children.

Several times the caregiver has seen Erica pinch the baby quite hard. She has also pushed the other two children over when they had a toy she wanted. She shouts a lot and likes to eat with her hands rather than use cutlery.

The caregiver becomes even more concerned one day when it became apparent that Erica's parents had been away for a long weekend and that the two children (Erica and her brother) had been left alone in the house for all of that time.

Learning activities II

1. What aspects of Erica's behaviour concern the caregiver?
2. What should the caregiver do when she finds the children have been left alone for 2 days?
3. Is this a case of suspected child abuse? Give reasons for your answer.

4. Find out about the child-protection legislation in your State or Territory.
5. What you would do if you were working with Alex or Erica. You might, if possible, discuss this with an experienced child-care professional or one of your teachers.

References

Australian Institute or Health and Welfare (1999). Child protection Australia 1997–98. Canberra, AIHW.

Australian National Training Authourity (1997). *CHC019: Accident prevention and child protection*. Melbourne, ACTRAC Products Ltd.

Birrel RG. (1968).The maltreatment syndrome in children: a hospital survey. *Med J Aust*, 2(23):1023–1029.

Briggs F, Hawkins R. (1997). *Child protection. A guide for teachers and child-care professionals*. Sydney, Allen and Unwin.

Kempe CH et al. (1962). The battered-child syndrome. *Journal of the American Medical Association* 22; 251(24):3288–3294.

National Child Protection Council *Preventing child abuse: A national strategy*. Sydney, NCPC.

Oates K, Donnelly AC. (1997). Influential papers in child abuse. *Child abuse and neglect*, 21(3):319–326.

Further reading

Briggs F. (1993). *Why my child?* Sydney, Allen and Unwin.

Clare C, Roe D. (1990). *Keeping our children safe*. Australian Early Childhood Association Resource Booklet, No.2. Canberra, AECA.

Goddard C. (1992). Child abuse: Understanding and responding. In Clements A, ed. *Infant and family health in Australia*. Melbourne, Churchill Livingstone.

National Association for the Prevention of Child Abuse and Neglect (NAPCAN) publications.

Pardeck JT. ed. (1989). *Child abuse and neglect: Theory, research and practice*. New York, Gordon and Breach.

Swan P. (1988). *Kids can say no! Kids have rights*. Redfern, Aboriginal Medical Service.

Tomison AM, Tucci J. (1997). *Emotional abuse: The hidden form of maltreatment*. Melbourne, National Child Protection Clearinghouse, No 8.

CHAPTER 10

Illness and other disorders in child care

THE AIM OF all health policies and practices within a child-care setting is to promote health and prevent illness. There will, however, be times when a child is unwell. There will also be children attending child-care who have health needs that require special attention and ongoing treatment. The caregiver has a responsibility to understand the specific health needs of each child and to provide the attention and treatment the child may require. Parents and health professionals will give details of this special care.

Health history

The past history and current health status of each child should be noted and recorded prior to admission into child care. These records form the basis of ongoing observations of each child and are valuable documents, as they will chart all ongoing health and developmental changes. Well kept records are part of the duty-of-care requirements and may be used as legal evidence if the need for this ever arose. Staff should also be aware of the ethical obligations of confidentiality regarding any information relating to a child and the family.

Type of information to be noted

- Any past illnesses or developmental concerns.
- Immunisation records.

- Any allergies.
- Any special health needs.
- Any current medication.
- Dietary preferences.
- Routine patterns and preferences of daily care.
- Social details.
- Contact details of parents.
- Emergency contact details.

Parents will also give written permission for urgent medical attention to be sought by child-care staff if the need for this ever arose.

Developing health policies

All child-care settings should have a written health policy that has been developed by parents and staff in conjunction with a health professional (who might be one of the parents). This policy should cover the general practices needed to promote health as well as emergency procedures (Principle 44 of the Accreditation Principles 1993). A thorough health policy document will include:

- Food and nutrition
- Immunisation
- Sun protection
- Accident prevention and safety
- Hygiene practices by staff and children
- Administration of medications to children
- Attendance of sick children and staff in the child-care setting
- Notification of the parents of sick children
- The separation of sick and well children in the child-care setting
- Recording of accidents to children and staff
- Fire emergency procedures
- Other emergency procedures.

Administration of prescribed medication

It is a professional requirement for staff to administer prescribed medicine to children. This is medicine that has been prescribed by a medical practitioner and dispensed by a pharmacist. The medicine container should be labelled with the name of the pharmacy and should include the name of the child. Medication may need to be given for a short period, as in the case of a short (acute) illness such as an infection, or over a long period as in the case of an ongoing condition (chronic) such as asthma.

Accurate written records must be kept of this procedure. A medicine book should be kept. A parent should complete the information regarding the medication each day. This information must include:

- Name of the child
- Name of medication
- Amount of medication to be given
- Route to be given—eg. by mouth, nasal spray, eye drops, local application to skin
- Way to be given—eg. syringe-type device, pipette, measuring spoon or cup
- Times to be given.

Before administering the medication the following should be checked by two staff members:

- Name of child on medication
- Name of medication
- Dose to be given
- Frequency of dose
- When last dose was given.

When giving the medication:

- Check the amount poured by holding the container at eye level.
- Pour the medication away from the label, as this prevents spills from staining and obscuring the label.
- Record that the medication has been given and sign with time of giving.
- Report if not all the medicine has been taken, such as when spitting out or spilling occurs.

Non-prescribed medication

There are many patent medicines available that can be bought over the counter in a chemist, supermarket or health food shop. The decision about whether child-care staff should administer such medicines would be made by parents, and staff response would reflect the philosophy of the service. Many child-care services have a policy that allows the administration of prescribed medication only. This protects the child-care service from giving the child inappropriate medication.

There is sometimes confusion regarding analgesics such as paracetamol. The use of such drugs should be kept to a minimum, but might be given in times of pain or fever if written permission stating that paracetamol could be administered under certain conditions had been given by the parents (and these conditions should be specified—eg. after immunisation). This sometimes happens at the time of enrolment. Some child-care settings would require that this permission be accompanied by a confirming note from a medical practitioner. Again, the decision regarding the use of accepted analgaesics should be made by the parents and staff and be part of the service's health policy.

Observation and assessment of health status

There are certain observations that help assess whether a child is unwell. The assessment is only useful if the child's normal condition is known. A child who is unwell presents with changes from her usual or normal condition.

- Skin

  How does the skin look? Is it clear or is there a rash or any infected patches? What colour is the skin? Is it pale, flushed, blotchy?

  How does the skin feel when you stroke the child? Is it dry, moist, sweaty, hot, cold, clammy?
- Eyes

  Are the eyes clear or are they red, swollen, sunken? Is there a discharge from the eyes?
- Ears and nose

  Is there a discharge from nostrils or ears? What is the discharge like? Is it clear, yellow, green or bloodstained? Is the child rubbing her ear?
- Breathing

  Is the breathing faster that normal? Is the child finding it hard to breathe? Can you hear wheezing or rattles? Does the child have a cough?
- Posture

  Is the child standing, sitting, lying as usual? Is there any sign of a stiff neck?
- Facial expression

  Does the child look relaxed and at ease? Does the facial expression show signs of pain or discomfort?
- Urine

  Is the child going to the toilet as usual, or more or less? What is the colour and smell of the urine?

- Faeces
  How many bowel actions is the child having? What is the colour and consistency of the faeces?
- Vomiting
  Is there any vomiting? How often is it occurring? What is the child vomiting? Is it undigested or half-digested food or greenish-yellow bile?
- Feeding and appetite
  Has this changed? Is the baby sucking well? (This is a very important sign—a baby who is not sucking is potentially very sick.)
  Did the child eat his snack or lunch? Is the child thirstier than usual?
- Activities and behaviour
  Is the child joining in activities as usual or is he quieter and less active? Is he much more active than usual and perhaps aggressive?
- Alertness
  Is the child as alert as usual or does he seem tired and listless?
- Sleep
  Is the child sleepier than usual or restless and unable to sleep?

Temperature, pulse and respiration rates

These measurements also give important information about whether a child is ill or well.

Temperature

A normal temperature for adults and children is 36–37° Celsius. The body reacts to infective organisms by an increase in temperature (ie. the child becomes febrile), which is a way of killing some of the organisms as well as increasing the white blood cell numbers for delivery to the parts of the body where they are needed. A temperature of more than 38°C is considered a fever.

An increase in body temperature is a sign that the child has an infection somewhere in the body. As a general rule, the higher the temperature the more serious is the infection. Taking a temperature within a child-care setting should be a simple procedure with a digital thermometer. The bulb of the thermometer should be placed under the arm and completely surrounded by skin and gently held in place for 3 minutes. This will give a reading that is accurate enough to establish whether the child has a fever. The temperature should never be taken rectally or orally within a child-care setting.

A fever together with other signs such as listlessness and loss of appetite are potentially serious and parents should be contacted so that immediate medical advice can be sought.

Pulse

This is the movement of the muscular artery wall as the blood is pumped in time with the heart. The beat can be felt wherever an artery goes over a bone or is close to the surface of the skin. The most common places to feel the pulse rate are:

- either temple, on the front side of the head;
- on either side of the neck, just down from the edge of the jaw;
- above the bone in the lower arm just up from the thumb.

A raised pulse rate is almost always accompanied by a raised body temperature. The pulse rate should always be measured when the person is resting, as activity alters the rate. The rate also differs with age and from person to person. The usual range for a resting pulse rate for the different age groups is:

Babies	95–160 per minute
Pre-schoolers	80–140 per minute
Adults	60–100 per minute.

Respiration rate

This is the number of times per minute that a person breathes in or out. The respiration rate varies with exercise and age and is also raised when there is a fever. It can be measured by gently placing a hand on the child's chest and counting the number of times the child breathes in over one minute. It should be counted when the child is at rest, and not immediately after exercise.

The usual range is:

Babies	30–60 per minute
Pre-schoolers	20–30 per minute
Adults	12–20 per minute.

Sick children and child care

This is one of the very difficult situations for which no satisfactory solution has yet been found. The young child who is attending a large group-care setting is much more likely to have frequent respiratory and middle ear infections than the child at home or in small group care. These children are not only infectious to other children and staff, they are generally febrile and miserable and need a gentle peaceful environment where they can be cared for by a familiar and loved person.

Many children remain unwell even when they are over the infectious stage of the illness. This sometimes causes conflict between parents and child-care staff. The family doctor considers the child to be non-infectious and writes a certificate, or tells the parents, that the child can officially return to child care. Yet the child is still not well enough to join in the daily program of activities and needs extra care and attention. This can cause a strain on already busy staff, who feel unable to meet the needs of the unwell child.

Ideally a parent, relative or close friend would care for the unwell child. Yet the structure of contemporary society often means that such a person is not freely available to care for a sick child. Young children generally attend child care because their parents are working and it may be difficult for either parent to take time off work each time a child is sick. The increase in the number of sole-parent families also means that the full responsibility for the care of sick children falls onto one parent.

A relative or close friend may not be available either. Grandparents have traditionally been the backstop for families, but many grandparents themselves now work and, in today's mobile society, they often live in other towns or States or even in other countries.

A possible solution would be to have a sickroom within the child-care setting with specific staff to care for sick children. However, this is very expensive and does not sit well with the current economic climate. Nor does this solution address the issue of trying to minimise the number of germs in a child-care setting. Children who are over the infectious period may be re-infected by other children.

Another suggested solution has been to have paid carers in the community who will take sick children into their own homes. This may not be the best for the emotional or developmental health of the sick child, who needs familiar people in familiar environments at this time. Sick-child-care programs have been tried in the United States and concern has been shown about the emotional aspects of such care.

There has been some acknowledgment at a government level of the difficulties faced by both parents and children. Official salary awards for paid sick leave now allow for a certain number of days to be used to care for sick children. This, however, only goes a short way to finding the solutions.

Assessing the sick child in child care

A sick child needs to be assessed in the same way as a child who has had an accident (Chapter 8). As a result of this assessment a decision would be made as to whether:

- Urgent medical or hospital attention should be sought and an ambulance called. This would happen in the case of severe shortness of breath, the lips becoming pale or blue, or any change in conscious state.
- The parents are called to immediately take the child to a medical practitioner or community health centre. This would happen when a baby under 6 months has fever or is not sucking well or has severe diarrhoea or vomiting. An older child who has a fever above 39°C should also be taken to a doctor.
- The parents are notified that the child is unwell and are requested to pick the child up as early as possible. This happens when a child is mildly unwell.

Caring for a sick child

There will be some situations where parents are unable to collect a child who is mildly unwell, and the child will need to stay at the child-care setting for several hours.

The child's condition will determine what care the child needs. A child who has a slight fever and is not hungry, but is drinking, will probably be best in a quiet area away from the other children where he can lie down, but look at books or be read to and do other quiet activities. Drinks should be frequently offered, as well as small frequent snacks, though the child should not be forced to eat. Lots of attention and reassurance should also be given.

Care should be taken to prevent any further cross-infection, even though in most illnesses the child would have been infectious before showing the first signs and symptoms.

Some common non-communicable illnesses in children

Asthma

Asthma is the most common cause of hospital admission in children and the rate of childhood asthma is increasing in Australia. In 1999 the Commonwealth Government identified asthma as a national health priority.

All child-care professionals at some time in their career will care for a child who is prone to asthma. It is important not only to have a general understanding of asthma and its treatment, but it is vital to have intimate knowledge of an individual child's history, ways the asthma presents and the necessary treatment. Some children will have mild asthma that is well controlled while others with moderate to severe asthma may need treatment while in child care.

Asthma is a condition where the lining of the airway passages going to the lungs becomes swollen, thus narrowing the space where the air needs to go. This makes it very difficult to breathe and the child becomes short of breath. There is often a wheezing sound as the child tries to breathe in and out. Not being able to breathe easily is very distressing and children are likely to become very anxious, which makes the shortness of breath much worse. Being short of breath can also cause the child to have problems with talking, which is a serious sign.

Causes of asthma

Asthma is usually triggered by something to which the airway is sensitive. These triggers include:

- respiratory infections;
- allergens such as dust mite, animals, pollens, moulds;
- cigarette smoke;
- exercise;
- sudden changes in climate;
- anxiety and emotional stress;
- drugs such as aspirin and some herbal and complementary medicines;
- chemical intolerance to substances found in foods (both natural and added);
- unknown factors.

Prevention and treatment

Removing the triggers

The best prevention is to keep the child and the triggers separate, though this is not always possible. Parents are encouraged, in consultation with health professionals, to develop an action plan which minimises the risks of asthma. This can include the removal of carpets and mats that tend to harbour dust mites. Children who are allergic to cats and dogs may need to choose a pet such as goldfish. Skin-prick tests will identify allergy to pollens. Swimming is less likely to trigger exercise-induced asthma than other physical activities and is also helpful for breathing exercises.

Medication

An action plan will also include advice regarding medication.

There are three main types of medication used in the prevention and treatment of an attack of asthma.

Relievers: These are broncho-dilating substances (eg. Ventolin, Respolin, Airomir, Asmol) that open up the airways and are used to reduce the severity of a threatened attack or to treat an episode once it has started. Relievers are given as an inhaled spray. It is important that any child who is prone to asthma has access to the prescribed bronchodilator puffer and space inhaler (spacer) at all times. It is a good idea for the child-care setting to keep spare reliever medication and a space inhaler in the first aid box.

Preventers: These are substances that reduce the inflammatory reaction of the body tissues, and are taken on a regular basis. They are often steroid-based and are usually taken by inhaled spray (eg. Aldecin, Becloforte, Becotide, Respocort). Non-steroidal preventers include Intal and Tildade.

The guidelines for the giving of the inhaled spray are the same as for any other medication. Young children will use space inhalers with a face mask (nebulisers are rarely used these days). Children should be sitting quietly while using a space inhaler. Staff should supervise the administration of the inhalation.

Older children will be able to use puffers, which require some breathing manipulation, provided they have been instructed in the correct technique by a parent, their doctor or an asthma educator. The use of puffers should be supervised within a child-care setting in order to ensure that the correct dose is taken.

Symptom controller medication: This medication (Serevent, Foradile, Oxis) may be used with children over 4 years of age where sleep is disturbed frequently by asthma symptoms. These children will be also taking regular preventer medication.

Treatment of asthma

Early treatment is important in order to reduce the severity of the attack. All episodes of asthma are potentially serious. Staff need to get to know what the early warning signs are in each individual child. Some older children will use a peak-flow meter, and a change in the measurements may give warning of a possible attack. Other general signs and symptoms are:

- shortness of breath and difficulty in breathing;
- wheezing sound when breathing in or out;
- a feeling of tightness in the chest;
- difficulty in talking.

Keeping the child quiet and calm is important, together with the immediate administration of a bronchodilator (reliever). The most comfortable position is usually sitting upright, with some support for the arms. The child should be reassured and closely observed.

With the spacer (with or without a face mask)

- shake inhaler and insert mouthpiece into spacer
- place spacer mouthpiece in child's mouth and fire one puff
- get the child to breathe in and out normally for about 4 breaths
- repeat in quick succession until 4 puffs have been given.

Without spacer (with older child)

- shake inhaler
- place mouthpiece in child's mouth. Fire one puff as the child inhales slowly and steadily
- ask child to hold that breath for 4 seconds and then take 4 normal breaths
- repeat until 4 puffs have been given.

A first attack of asthma

- if a child collapses or appears to have difficulty breathing, CALL AN AMBULANCE IMMEDIATELY.
- give 4 puffs every 4 minutes until the ambulance arrives
- remember that no harm is likely to result from giving a reliever drug to someone who does not have asthma (National Asthma Campaign 2000).

Communication with parents

This is a very important part of preventing asthma attacks. Parents should ensure that the child-care setting has all the details of the child's asthma. These details can be provided on set forms that list known triggers, signs and symptoms and specify immediate treatment.

More informal ongoing communication on a day-to-day basis means that both staff and parents know what has happened during the day and while the child is at home. This knowledge may well help to prevent an attack of asthma.

The Asthma Foundation in each State and Territory (see Chapter 12) has community educators who give in-service programs to children's services, as do some local health authorities.

The National Asthma Campaign has developed a 3+ Visit Plan for general practitioners which ensures that children with asthma have medical supervision. Parents of children with asthma could be encouraged to ask their general practitioners about this treatment plan.

Diabetes mellitus (sugar diabetes)

There are two types of diabetes, though children only have Type 1.

- Type 1 (insulin-dependent) needs to be controlled with insulin. It often starts in childhood, though not often before about 4 or 5 years of age.
- Type 2 (non-insulin dependent) can be controlled by diet and starts well into adult life. It is often associated with poor diet and being very overweight.

Insulin-dependent diabetes in children

Insulin is a hormone produced in the pancreas, which controls the use of all glucose in the body (see Endocrine system, Chapter 4). If there is little or no insulin being produced, the glucose that has been absorbed into the blood stream (glucose is the end result of all carbohydrates that have been eaten) cannot be used and concentrates in the blood and urine. The person gets tired and sick, is constantly thirsty, and passes a lot of urine, and the urine, breath and sweat smell sweet. Untreated, this condition could lead to coma and death.

The treatment is to give insulin and control the carbohydrate intake, so that the amount of insulin given will balance the carbohydrate eaten. To do this in children and get the balance right can sometimes be challenging. Children are active and growing, so their carbohydrate needs vary, which means their insulin needs also vary.

Insulin can only be given by injection under the skin, so the child needs to start learning how to do this himself. Of course, this calls for help and support from family, and health professionals. Regular measurements need to be taken of blood sugar levels and of the amount of sugar in the urine in order to ascertain whether the diabetes is being controlled.

Child-care professionals play an important role in supporting both the child with diabetes and the family. This support is given by finding out about diabetes and how it affects the child. Parent support organisations can be good sources of information and will often send information packs to child-care centres. Ensuring that the correct diet is given at the correct time, and noting if the child seems unwell, are all important aspects of care.

Complications of diabetes

Low blood sugar

One of the dangers with diabetes is that if the correct amount of food is not taken after insulin is given, then the child's blood sugar levels will become too low (hypoglycaemia). This can happen if a snack or meal is too late or the child is not well and misses some food. It can also happen if the child expends an unusual amount of energy.

Low blood sugar in a child who has diabetes is a potentially dangerous condition. The child will initially become pale and sweaty, may become irrational and aggressive, and could become unconscious. In the worst situation a child with very low blood sugar can quickly become unconscious and go into a hypoglycaemic coma. This can happen very quickly. It is imperative that the blood sugar be immediately raised and this is done by giving some fast-acting sugar, such as a sweet drink (lemonade) or jelly babies, before the child's conscious state is altered.

The child-care professional needs to be very observant regarding this child. All snacks and meals should be given on time, any not eaten should be noted and supplements given in place of the uneaten food. Close communication with parents will ensure that all important information regarding diet and supplements will be known. New and relief child-care staff must be adequately briefed before working with the child.

High blood sugar

High blood sugar levels (hyperglycaemia) can also lead to coma, though this happens much more slowly than in the case of hypoglycaemia. High blood sugar levels occur when the diabetes is not well controlled, such as when the insulin dose is too low for the amount of carbohydrate the child is eating or when the child eats foods, such as sweets or cakes, that are not allowed on the diet. The child will need to seek medical attention and may well be hospitalised in order to get the dose of insulin right and the diet balanced.

The long-term dangers of uncontrolled diabetes in childhood are severe complications in adult life. These complications include heart disease, kidney disease, blindness and problems with blood circulation, which can lead to loss of limbs.

Responsibility of the child-care professional

Is it hypo- or hyperglycaemia?

Some child-care staff are concerned about how to tell the difference between hypoglycaemia and hyperglycaemia. All physical and behavioural changes that come on quickly in a child with diabetes should be treated as low blood sugar and SUGAR GIVEN IMMEDIATELY in the form of a sweet or a sugary drink. It is a good idea for staff to keep sweets at hand for such a situation.

Parties and celebrations

Children with diabetes have a diet that allows no sweet foods, which all too often form the basis of parties and celebratory occasions. Think of Easter and all the chocolate consumed by both adults and children! It is important that the child with diabetes is taught what he is, and what he is not, allowed to eat and that supervision is in place with the younger child.

Having a child with diabetes in a group can be a bonus for the diets of all children and provide challenges for staff to provide exciting food with a low sugar content. Discussions with a community dietitian can provide ideas for such foods. There are also publications available from the Diabetes Association that give recipes for foods suitable for diabetics.

Diabetes education

The Diabetes Association (see Chapter 12) is a community non-government organisation that gives support to families who have children (or adults) with diabetes. Staff of the Diabetes Association are available to talk to staff in child-care settings.

It is important that other children also understand what is happening to the diabetic child. There are story books available for children of all ages. These books explain diabetes, using real characters, and not only give information but also provide reassurance that a normal active life is what should be expected.

Epilepsy

Although this is not a common condition, it is useful for the caregiver to have a general understanding of the forms of epilepsy.

Epilepsy is a condition where the electrical activity of the brain gets out of control and causes altered consciousness and/or a fit (or seizure) to occur. There can be uncontrollable muscle movements with sharp jerking movements, and sometimes loss of bowel and bladder muscle control.

Sometimes a child will become prone to epileptic fits after a head injury or infection such as meningitis where brain damage has occurred. There is, however, often no known cause for a person's epilepsy. There are several forms of epilepsy:

- *Grand mal,* where there is often a warning that the fit is likely to occur. The child may show disrupted behaviour and then fall to the ground, jerking uncontrollably. A loss of consciousness nearly always occurs and sometimes the tongue may be bitten. The child will often urinate and/or defecate during the fit. After the fitting stops the child may remain unconscious for several minutes and be quite confused and sleepy upon awakening.

- *Petit mal*, where the episode may go almost unnoticed. The conscious state is altered though the child does not usually fall. The child most usually stops what he is doing and stares blankly into space for up to 20 seconds.

What to do during a grand mal fit

Keeping the child safe is the main consideration. Do not attempt to move or control the child's movements, but move furniture and other children out of the way. Observe the child closely and place him on his side (coma position) when the fitting has stopped. Reassure the child when he becomes conscious. Older children become very embarrassed by the loss of bowel and bladder control and need sympathetic support and care.

Parents will need to be contacted and told the child has had a fit. If this is the first fit a child has had, then immediate medical attention should be sought. Parents will also make a medical appointment for a child for whom this is not the first fit, so that the child and his treatment can be assessed.

Any child who remains unconscious for more than 3–5 minutes should be immediately taken to hospital by ambulance. The child-care setting should have a policy that covers such eventualities.

What to do during a petit mal episode

Sitting quietly with the child is usually all that can be done in this situation. The child will not remember anything about the blank period and could be a little confused. Talking quietly with the child will reassure her. She may wish to rest, but allow her to decide when she will join in the group activities again. It would be advisable for her not to engage in strenuous physical activities immediately after a petit mal episode. Her parents will also need to be told at the end of the day that a petit mal episode occurred. This, too, should be documented in the child's records.

Triggers of epileptic fits

Most times the triggers are unknown, though infection, tiredness and emotional stress are all recognised as causes. Flashing or flickering lights can cause epileptic episodes to occur. These flashing lights can be from the television or from sunshine flickering between trees. Seven hundred children in Japan were taken to hospital with epileptic-type episodes in

December 1997 after watching a television cartoon where one of the characters had flashing red eyes. Strobe lights at children's parties are also best avoided.

Treatment

Avoiding known triggers is an important preventive measure. The standard medical treatment is anticonvulsant therapy, which is usually a combination of drugs taken in tablet form. Sometimes these drugs make a child sleepy, so it may take some time to get the balance right between preventing fits and not having a sleepy child. The observations of child-care professionals are invaluable in helping to get the balance right. Drug therapy needs to be changed as the child gets older. Adolescence may also be a time where extra care needs to be taken to control the epilepsy.

Long-term outlook

This is generally very good in the case of children who do not have underlying brain damage. Some forms of epilepsy do not require treatment after adolescence. Others will need ongoing anticonvulsant therapy to control the condition and prevent fits.

It is important that children with epilepsy are encouraged to do all the same activities as the other children. This includes swimming though, as with all children, staff need to observe and supervise the child closely.

Infantile febrile convulsions

A sudden rise in temperature in a baby or young child can trigger a convulsion, which is a type of fit. The baby may initially stiffen or even lose consciousness and then begin to twitch all over the body. The eyes may roll back. Any baby or child who has such an episode should be seen immediately by a doctor. Urgent hospital treatment is needed if the child has been unconscious for more than 5 minutes or does not immediately regain consciousness.

Brain damage can occur as a result of a prolonged febrile convulsion, so it is very important to reduce a baby's or child's temperature in order to prevent a convulsion. Keeping the child cool by the use of tepid washes, taking off clothes and cooling the room are measures that can be taken. Paracetamol can also be given.

Remember that medical advice should be sought if a baby under 6 months of age has a raised temperature of any degree.

Infantile eczema

This is a very itchy skin rash that is often scaly and weepy. Eczema commonly occurs on the front of the arms and legs, the face and scalp and the trunk. The cause is usually unknown, although children with eczema often have family members who had eczema as children and now have allergies or asthma. Some young children who have eczema develop asthma or hay fever as they get older.

The extreme itchiness is the main problem, as the child naturally wants to scratch the rash. The scratching then breaks the skin and micro-organisms get in, causing an infection. Treatment aims to control the symptoms by reducing the itchiness and preventing infection.

- Cotton clothing should be worn, as this is cooler on the itchy skin.
- Finger nails should be kept very short and clean, as this helps to prevent breaking the skin and introducing infection when scratching.
- The child should be prevented from becoming too hot, as heat increases the itch.
- The itch can be reduced by applications of prescribed creams. Hydrocortisone cream is often used and this reduces the inflammatory reaction of the rash.

Other less common conditions

Coeliac disease

This is a genetic disease that causes an inability to digest gluten, which is found in wheat, rye, barley and oats. The child with coeliac disease is unable to have foods made from these products and the cereal intake must come from rice and maize (sweet corn) foods. There is no cure for coeliac disease; the disease is controlled by a life-long gluten-free diet.

The first symptoms usually occur after the child has started solids. Bowel actions are especially offensive in smell and the child often stops gaining weight or even loses weight.

Cystic fibrosis (also mentioned in Chapter 3)

This is another genetic disease. Mucus builds up in the respiratory passages, causing serious chest infections. Cystic fibrosis also prevents the pancreas from secreting adequate amounts of enzymes needed for the digestion of food. The child is therefore unable to absorb food, has diarrhoea and fails to thrive.

In earlier times, children who had cystic fibrosis died when quite young but the outlook has improved with modern treatment and most children now live well into adulthood. There are replacement enzymes available that help with absorption of food from the small intestine, and antibiotics to treat chest infections. Intensive physiotherapy helps prevent chest infections.

Environmental concerns

Many poisonous substances, both natural and synthetic, exist in the environment. Some plants such as foxgloves and oleander are poisonous. Many metals are poisonous.

Children and lead poisoning

Lead is a toxic metal that has been of concern since Roman times when people were poisoned by drinking water that came through lead pipes.

Even mild lead poisoning is of concern in children because their bodies absorb the lead much more easily than adults. Lead poisoning can have harmful effects on child development and can lead to intellectual disabilities. Other symptoms can include tiredness, headache, abdominal pain and anaemia. Behavioural changes are also common.

How does lead poisoning occur?

We may not use lead pipes any more but there are many other sources of lead in our enviroment.

Some of the sources are:

- Air pollution through the fumes of cars using leaded petrol. The introduction of non-leaded fuel for cars will, over time, help reduce the amount of lead in the air.
- Paint in the past contained lead and this was a common cause of poisoning. The renovation of old houses can cause old lead paint to be exposed and to become airborne in the house dust.
- Soil in some industrial areas contains lead. Port Pirie in South Australia is situated near a lead smelter and the soil was found to contain high levels of lead. In other areas the soil may become contaminated by industrial waste containing flaking paint or the solid waste from leaded fuel.
- Food grown in contaminated soil will contain lead.
- Cooking pots which are finished with a lead-based glaze or are made of a metal which contains lead.

Lead poisoning can also be passed from the mother to the fetus *in utero*. A mother who works or lives in an environment where there is lead contamination may not show signs of the poisoning herself but the lead levels in her body may harm the fetus.

How can lead poisoning be prevented in children?

All parents and professionals should have information about the dangers of lead poisoning. The main aim is to prevent poisoning occurring in the first place, which means the elimination of environmental hazards. Government legislation regarding lead free fuel is one such example. Awareness of the dangers of airborne lead particles and taking safety measures when renovating buildings is another example.

Blood lead levels in Australian children do seem to be getting lower, probably due to the reduction of leaded petrol (AIHW 2000). However, it is still suggested that young children (9 months to 5 years) who live in high risk environments should have their blood lead levels regularly assessed.

Behavioural concerns

Children's behaviour often changes, and needs to be viewed within a developmental, cultural and social context. Adult expectations of children and their behaviour can be unrealistic.

It would be misjudging a child of 20 months to say her behaviour was a problem because she was unwilling to share her toys and kept snatching things from other children. Developmentally a child of this age has little or no concept of sharing, and the social and physical environment should take this into account. There should be enough equipment for all children and the area should be set up so that there is enough space for each child not to feel overwhelmed or crowded.

A 3–4-year-old who is not given a choice of appropriate challenging activities may become bored and consequently disruptive. This is not a behavioural problem but rather a failure to acknowledge the wide-ranging developmental needs of a child of that age.

An 8-year-old who breaks a house window while playing cricket with friends in the backyard may well be a budding cricketer. She really needs a bigger space than a suburban backyard, rather than being considered to have done something wrong.

Behavioural disorders

Behavioural disorders are not as easy to describe or diagnose as a physical illness. In a physical condition, such as diabetes, there is a definite list of signs and symptoms, and tests can be done to check blood sugar levels. These measurements are used to confirm the diagnosis.

There are certainly descriptions of behavioural disorders that list the signs and symptoms. Psychological tests are also available to assess certain aspects of a child's behaviour and personality, and how he functions in certain situations. The very different personalities of children and the different social and emotional environments in which they are raised have sometimes made it difficult to decide upon an exact diagnosis.

Autism

This condition is classified as an emotional and social developmental disorder. The child may have problems in all forms of communication, social interaction, emotional attachment and play activities. There is also an apparent inability to empathise or understand the feelings of others.

Autism is usually recognised between 18 months and 3 years of age. Children at these ages are starting to socialise with others, and to take on other personalities during dramatic play. The child with autism is unable to engage in social activities or in dramatic play, and may be totally passive and withdrawn.

There is no single known cause for autism but is thought that it is linked to brain development and to genetic and environmental factors. Autism is four times more common in boys than in girls.

Some children have only some of the signs of autism. Terms such as 'pervasive development disorder' or 'autism spectrum disorder' are often used in such situations.

Children with autism are often integrated into mainstream children's services. There will be links with psychologists and other allied health workers. A supplementary special needs worker may also be employed to assist with a specific programs of activities for these children.

Attention Deficit Hyperactivity Disorder (ADHD)

There have always been children who have been so active that they have caused disruption to themselves and their families. In the past, these children have been loosely described as hyperactive or hyperkinetic. More recently it was observed that some children had problems with concentration or attending to a task for any length of time. This became known as Attention Deficit Disorder (ADD).

Current thinking is that hyperactivity and attention deficit often go together and so the group of behaviours has become known as Attention Deficit Hyperactivity Disorder (ADHD). This disorder has received much attention in developed countries since the 1980s.

There has also been much debate about whether ADHD exists as a specific disorder and, if it does, if it is being over-diagnosed (or not being diagnosed enough). There are certainly geographical differences in the number of children being diagnosed with ADHD. The diagnosis of ADHD is made much more frequently in the United States than in the United Kingdom (Valman 1997) and, within Australia, more in New South Wales than in Victoria (Swan 1995). There is no reason to think that children in New South Wales are different from those of the same age and social backgrounds in Victoria. There are certainly some cultural differences between children in the United Kingdom and those in the United States, but is that enough to explain why one group has much less ADHD than the other?

It has been suggested that the main differences between all these geographical areas is whether ADHD is accepted by paediatricians as a 'real' disorder or not. So, some people say, the difference in the rates of ADHD is due to the medical education and attitude of the doctors rather than to any real differences in the children's behaviour. This debate is still going on. What is known is that more boys are diagnosed with ADHD than girls. This is similar to the difference in accident rates between boys and girls.

How to recognise ADHD

Most children at times are boisterous, very energetic and may jump from one activity to another, which can be very tiring for adults. Many children at one time or another are:

- unable to concentrate;
- show poor short-term memory;
- extremely restless;
- very excitable and impulsive;
- destructive;
- disruptive;
- accident prone;
- irritable and aggressive;
- experiencing problems with learning.

Further investigation should take place if a child shows many of these behaviours most of the time.

It may be that the child has ADHD, but there are many other reasons for a child having the behaviours described above. These possible causes should be eliminated before a diagnosis is made.

Psycho-social environment

This includes an assessment of the psychological and social environment of the child.

- A child is likely to be restless if she lives in an overcrowded flat with inadequate playing space and where she can't get outside to run or climb.
- A child who plays in unsafe areas with unsafe equipment will have accidents.
- A child who wakes up to the television blaring or loud music playing, and whose routine in the morning is inconsistent and generally rushed, is likely to be very restless before he gets to child-care or to school.
- A child who has no clear limits set for her will be impulsive, due to having no guidelines regarding what behaviour is acceptable.
- A child whose care is inconsistent and of poor quality can become destructive and aggressive.
- A child who does not have enough appropriate activities may behave in a disruptive way.
- Family disruption may also cause the child to become restless. Events such as illness, parental disagreements, separation or divorce are not uncommon disruptions to children's lives.

Biological concerns

- Hearing impairment can make a child restless and unable to concentrate on any one activity for any length of time. Learning may also be difficult for this child.
- A mild degree of intellectual disability or brain damage may also cause a child to be restless and show other symptoms similar to ADHD.
- Fetal alcohol syndrome also contributes to behaviours that are very similar to ADHD.
- Other physical illnesses can disturb a child's behaviour.

Diagnosing ADHD

The ways that diseases or disorders are diagnosed should be similar, whether they be physical or behavioural. For example, a child who has diabetes will show certain physical signs and symptoms that match what is known about diabetes. Being able to measure the blood sugar levels is one of the important diagnostic points.

It should be possible to diagnose ADHD in the same way, ie. to have a list of signs and symptoms that match what is known about the disorder. There should also be a test (or tests) available that confirm if the child has ADHD.

As ADHD becomes more accepted as a recognised disorder, more work has been done on formalising the diagnosis. A list of behaviours (or signs and symptoms) that are thought to be criteria for diagnosing ADHD has been developed. Parents and teachers, as well as paediatricians, are involved in completing these lists. The National Health and Medical Research Council (NHMRC 1996) has reviewed the current literature and published assessment and management advice for health and allied professionals.

Treating ADHD

The current accepted form of treatment is a combination of medication and behaviour therapy which are generally used together. The medication used to treat ADHD is an amphetamine which, although it is a stimulant, calms the child down. Some children who do not respond to stimulants may be given anti-depressants. It should be remembered that both stimulants and anti-depressants restore chemical balance to brain function, which is what the child with ADHD needs.

Behaviour therapy aims to help parents and caregivers as well as the child. Children and/or families may have regular sessions with a psychologist or other professional who will discuss ways of guiding the child's behaviour with the parents and caregivers. Consistency of guidance is important so there is ongoing co-operation between the child and all those concerned with his treatment.

Diet

Many parents are unwilling to have their children take amphetamines and feel that ADHD is caused by food additives or an intolerance to certain foods. There is, as yet, no real evidence that this is the case, however it can be a positive measure to eliminate certain foods from a child's diet as long as the diet remains nutritionally well balanced. Many of the eliminated foods are often in the form of artificial food colourings found in sweets and soft drinks. The child who is on a special diet will also receive a lot of attention and this, too, is positive. A combination of a well balanced, nutritious diet together with plenty of positive attention can only be beneficial. Care should be taken that children are not put onto 'fad' diets that eliminate essential foods, so advice should be taken to ensure that the diet is well balanced.

The child in hospital

In the past, hospitalisation was a most traumatic experience for young children, as parents and other familiar persons were discouraged from staying with their child. This meant that the child was in a strange, fearful place where painful things happened and where they felt totally abandoned by their family. The emotional stress made the physical pain much harder to bear.

Happily, hospital experiences for young children these days are much less traumatic even if they are not always pleasant. Many minor operations can be done as a day procedure and the child need not have to stay in hospital overnight. With longer hospital stays, parents are encouraged to stay and assist with the daily routines such as bathing and feeding, and to provide ongoing emotional care. Appropriate activities are also provided for the children. These activities can help the child to express through play their feelings about what is happening to them in the hospital.

Child-care professionals sometimes work in hospitals developing play programs and working directly with the hospitalised children. These programs are as much part of the overall health care as are medical and nursing care.

Child-care settings can provide an opportunity for children to learn more about hospitals. Dramatic activities simulating hospital play can be set up in the home corner, stories about being in hospital can be read to the children, and staff from hospitals can come to the child-care centre.

Sometimes children regress and their behaviour after a stay in hospital becomes that of a younger child. The young child may want a bottle again, or wet the bed or cling to parents and not want to come back to child care. This regression to an earlier stage of behaviour needs to be accepted without question while the child has time to recover from the hospital experience.

Rachel is 3 years old and has a benign tumour on her bowel that needs to be removed. Her parents have taken her to the surgeon, who has arranged to be operate on Rachel in a month's time. It is expected that Rachel will need to be in hospital for 1–2 days . She will need a general anaesthetic and will have stitches and a dressing over the wound. It is expected that she will not feel very much pain, but it will hurt her to move. The surgeon has recommended that Rachel be admitted to a children's hospital, where the staff are specially trained to care for children.

Rachel's parents know that this is not going to be a pleasant experience but they want to make it as untraumatic as they can. The nurse in the surgeon's room has given them some articles about preparing Rachel for hospital and says to call her if they have more questions.

Continued

Next day they discuss Rachel's forthcoming hospitalisation with the director and staff of the child-care centre that Rachel attends full-time. They find it is reassuring to share their concern about Rachel's operation. The staff at the child-care centre have just had an in-service about the role of dramatic play in preparing children for elective surgery, and have lots of ideas to help prepare Rachel.

The child-care staff plan to include hospital play in the program. They start by having some story books about children in hospitals and slowly develop the theme by putting out hospital equipment such as bowls and kidney dishes in the home corner. They also find some posters about children in hospitals and put these up on the wall. Next week they add some stethoscopes, plastic syringes (without needles), gowns and masks to the play and start discussing hospital procedures more directly. Other children share their hospital experiences and there is an impromptu showing of scars, both old and new, some large and some so small they can scarcely be seen. The staff respond to all the children very seriously and respectfully.

Rachel has a favourite teddy and her parents put some elastoplast tape on his abdomen to become part of the dramatic play in the child-care centre. Many of the children join in putting teddy to bed and operating on his tummy. One of the children who had recently been to hospital takes over the role of anaesthetist and describes in great detail how teddy is being put to sleep. Another child cuddles teddy after the operation and makes comforting sounds.

Rachel's parents took her to hospital the night before the operation. The ward was full of other children, just as in the stories about hospital she had read. Her mother stayed with her, and so did her teddy. The nurses liked the elastoplast on teddy and said she could take him with her in the morning. Rachel was prepared for her operation next morning.

The operation went well and Rachel's mother was still there when she woke up. There were also lots of people wearing the sort of masks they had played with at child-care. Rachel had a strip of elastoplast over her abdomen just like teddy, though she felt very sleepy and didn't feel like talking about it.

Rachel got better very quickly and went home the next day. She had to go back to the surgeon a week later and the nurse took the stitches out of Rachel's and teddy's tummy. It felt funny, but didn't hurt. Next week Rachel went back to child care and showed them all her scar. She even still had marks around the scar where the stitches had been.

Continued

Rachel was glad to be out of hospital and back at child care. She hugged her mother very hard, though, and needed reassurance that she would be picked up in the afternoon. Rachel's mother hugged her back and told her that she'd be there after afternoon snack time. A caregiver quietly took Rachel's hand and held it until Rachel was ready to go and play.

Learning activities

1. Observe four children and note their appearance relating to health.
2. Discuss the health policies of your children's service with the Director.
3. Find out as much as you can about Diabetes Australia and the Asthma Foundation (see Chapter 12).
4. Visit the children's section of your local library and see if you can find children's books relating to any of the conditions in this chapter.

References

Australian Institute of Health and Welfare (2000). Australia's health 2000: the seventh biennial health report of the Australian Institute and Welfare. Canberra, AIHW.

Commonwealth of Australia (1993). *Putting children first: Quality improvement and accreditation system handbook*. Sydney, National Child Care Accreditation Council.

Green C, Chee K. (1997). *Understanding ADHD: A parent's guide to attention deficit hyperactivity disorder in children*. London, Vermillion.

National Asthma Campaign (2000). *First aid for asthma*. Melbourne, National Asthma Campaign. This is a wall chart which can be obtained free of charge from the National Asthma Campaign (see Chapter 12 for contact details).

National Health and Medical Research Council (1996). *Attention Deficit Hyperactivity Disorder*, Canberra, AGPS.

Swan N. (1995). Four Corners program on ADHD. Sydney, Australian Broadcasting Corporation.

Further reading

Asthma Australia publications.

Association for Welfare of Children in Hospitals publications.

Braithwaite A. (1991). *I have diabetes*. London, Dinosaur.

Diabetes Australia publications.

Leach P. (1991). *The parents' A to Z: A guide to children's health, growth and happiness*. Harmondsworth, Penguin.

National Asthma Campaign publications.

Valman B. (1998). *Children's symptoms*. Australian Medical Association edition. Sydney, Dorling Kindersley.

Recommended viewing

Swan N. (1995). Four Corners program ADHD. Sydney, Australian Broadcasting Corporation.

CHAPTER 11

Occupational health and safety

WORK IS IMPORTANT to most people. Not only does it provide an income, there is the satisfaction of having a career and of achieving aims. Work can also be an important part of social life. Many lifelong friendships initially started at work.

Yet work can also be a threat to health. Every year people are seriously injured and a number actually die in their workplace. There are different threats in different types of work. Jobs such as mining and those in the construction and building industry may present physical hazards. Jobs in the human services are often mentally exhausting.

Work in children's services, like many of the other caring professions, such as nursing, makes both physical and mental demands. We have concentrated throughout this book on the health of children and their families. Let us now look at the health of caregivers.

It is the right of all workers to be kept safe and well in the workplace. Employers and employees need to work together to make this happen. Both groups have rights and responsibilities towards having a healthy and safe workplace.

Legal responsibilities

There are legal requirements governing occupational health and safety throughout Australia. Overall legislation relates to work places in general and each profession and industry has specific regulations relating to their type of work.

It is the employer's responsibility to provide and maintain a safe and healthy working environment. It is the employee's responsibility to follow all instructions relating to keeping the environment safe and healthy.

Christa and Joe work for a mobile play group that operates from a small bus and visits several sites around their metropolitan area. They stop at a long-term caravan site, a church hall and a park each week. There are always lots of children and parents at each site.

Christa and Joe enjoy their work though they find packing and unpacking the bus the most tedious part. They especially dislike Friday afternoons when all the equipment has to be unpacked and stored in a shed over the weekend. None of the pieces of equipment is really heavy but items such as parts of mobile climbing equipment are very bulky and need two people to handle them. The occupational health and safety policy of the mobile service states that two people must be used when handling this equipment.

Here we have a situation where the employer has taken the safety of the employees into consideration by stating that two people are always needed to lift the bulky pieces of equipment. It is the responsibility of the employees to obey the regulations at all times.

One Friday Christa and Joe arrived back to unpack the bus when Joe was called to the phone. He was a long time away and Christa, who needed to pick her two children up from school, was in a hurry. She decided to start unpacking the equipment by herself. She found the larger pieces difficult and tripped over, falling heavily to the ground. She was found to have broken her ankle and was unable to work for four weeks.

In this situation, the employee has not followed the instructions of the employer, had put herself at risk and been injured.

Workers' compensation

All States and Territories have laws which require the employer to take out insurance against employees being injured at work. These schemes are known by such terms as Workhealth or Workcover and are administered by government authorities.

Duty of care

This is a term which you will frequently hear when discussing occupational health and safety issues. It is a legal term and refers to the responsibilities of both employer and employee in keeping themselves, the children and the environment healthy and safe.

In the case of Christa, it might be found that she had breached her duty of care responsibilities because she ignored the clear instructions of her employer. It could also be found that her employer had breached duty of care by not having an extra person to help when Joe was called away.

Care of employees

The aim of occupational health and safety legislation and practices is to prevent accidents in the workplace. However, there are legal safeguards to protect employees if an accident does occur in the workplace.

Workers' compensation may provide payment to workers to cover lost wages and medical expenses. It is not an automatic payment. The accident must be immediately reported to the appropriate authorities and compensation claimed. The claim will be examined and evidence sought from such sources as employers and medical experts, before a ruling on compensation is given.

There are cases where an accident at work prevents the employee from continuing in that profession. Workers' compensation may also include funds for re-training in another career.

Trade unions and professional associations

Each industry has a union or association which helps to maintain and promote workers' rights and conditions. This includes the right to a safe working environment and unions are represented on government committees which draw up occupational health and safety legislation.

Reporting of incidents

It is very important that any untoward incident at work be reported and recorded in the Accident Book. This applies equally to minor incidents as well as major accidents because of the risk of later complications.

Rhia works with the 3–5 year olds and is chatting with them in the sandpit. Everyone is very busy building roads which requires moving sand around in wheelbarrows at the edge of the sandpit. One of the younger children takes a wheelbarrow to a path and some sand is spilt. Rhia goes to help sweep it up and slips over. She falls to the ground but on getting up doesn't seem to have hurt herself. She shakes the sand from her clothes and reassures her colleagues she is fine. The incident is not recorded in the Accident Book.

Two weeks later Rhia finds her right knee is very stiff and seems a little swollen. She visits her General Practitioner whose first question is whether she has recently fallen.

Rhia may need to take time off work and she would be eligible for Worker's Compensation for a work-related injury. This is now going to be much more difficult as there is no written record of the initial accident.

Keeping the workplace healthy and safe

Without appropriate precautions, child care can be quite hazardous for employees. Infections, injury through lifting and handling of chemicals such as bleach for cleaning, and the stress of a very demanding (even if rewarding) job are some potential dangers.

These dangers can be minimised by employers and employees working together to recognise the hazards and to plan preventive practices. All workplaces should have an occupational health and safety policy and a nominated staff member who is responsible for seeing that these policies become practice. Some large organisations will have a Health and Safety Committee.

Let us look at some of the potential hazards in child care.

Infections

In Chapter 5, we looked in detail at how easily infection spreads in childcare. Infection does not spread only between the children, but also between children and staff. Being exposed to infectious diseases is an occupational hazard in childcare.

Employers must develop policies and guidelines that help to minimise cross infection. Employees should follow the infection control guidelines. It is also the responsibility of the employer to provide information regarding immunisation and other preventive programs. This is all discussed in Chapter 5.

General health

Caregivers have to be alert and responsive to children's needs at all times. This requires a high level of fitness and general health. Healthy staff are able to care for themselves as well as the children. Staying healthy means having a well balanced diet and plenty of exercise, rest and relaxation away from work. Personal life-style is also important. Serious personal and work problems can occur through alcohol abuse and drug use.

Stress

Caring for children can be one of the most enjoyable and positive careers. It can also, on a day to day basis, be very stressful.

Kay has completed a Diploma of Children's Services and has been working as a group leader in the 2–3-year-olds' room at a large long-day care centre in the outer suburbs. The area is relatively new and there are a lot of young families. There is also some government emergency housing where families in crisis are placed short-term. The child-care centre has an arrangement with the local government council to keep some places available for the children of these families.

Kay works in her room with three other staff members: one has a Certificate in Child Care and the other two are untrained (Level 1) though they have much experience. It is always busy in her room especially on Monday morning. This particular Monday morning, one of the Level 1 workers has rung in to say she is sick. Kay feels rather annoyed as this is the third Monday in a row that this has happened, and last week the Director had problems finding relief staff.

Teng is attending the centre for the first time this morning. His mother brought him in very early. She could not stay with him as she had an urgent medical appointment. Teng is very distressed and Kay is finding it hard to comfort him.

The parents naturally all want to talk with Kay as they bring the children in. She also wants to listen to them as she thinks it is important to share family events and experiences. All children who come to child care are part of a family and Kay tries, as much as possible, to provide an environment which reflects what happens in the family.

Let's look at Kay and her situation. It is half past nine on a Monday morning. She started work at half past seven and spent the first half hour setting up the indoor and outdoor areas with help from another staff member. This is hard physical work requiring bending and lifting. At eight o'clock Kay received the message about the unwell staff member, which caused her to feel anxious about having enough staff for the day. She was also concerned that the relief staff member may not know the children, which makes it hard for both the children and the other staff. Then Teng arrived and his mother hurriedly left. Kay sat with Teng comforting him and trying to chat with parents as she did so. She feels distressed about Teng and knows his mother has recently separated from her partner and is living in emergency accommodation. This accommodation is only temporary, so Teng may soon have many other changes in his life.

Kay is not alone in experiencing these stresses and she does plan her life to fit in with the demands of child care and her own personal needs.

Kay has adequate sleep and feels fresh and alert in the mornings, having eaten breakfast before coming to work. At work she makes sure that she takes her breaks regularly. The staff room is light and airy and she relaxes with the newspaper or a magazine. She sometimes walks to a nearby park at lunch time and sits on a bench in the shade looking at the pattern made by the leaves in the sunlight.

A couple of evenings each week, Kay plays netball with a local club. She enjoys the physical exercise and company. She also enjoys the fun and competition of the games although she doesn't mind too much if her team loses. She often has a meal at an Italian restaurant with her team mates after the match. They usually have pasta and salad.

Kay walks with a friend on the other evenings. She lives in a suburb which has access to a small tract of bushland and she finds the sounds and smells of the birds and gum trees relaxing. The walk keeps her physically fit.

At home, Kay enjoys reading and watching some television. She lives with her boyfriend, who appreciates the demands of her work. He shares all the housework and cooking. They go to the pub with friends at the weekend but more for the socialising than the drinking.

Kay recognises at work that she is feeling annoyed with the staff member who has been calling in sick on Mondays. She talks about her feelings with the Director and together they decide to gently discuss the matter with the staff member and to try to find a positive solution.

Physical hazards

Falls, tripping and slipping

There are always toys and other equipment on the indoor floors and outdoor ground areas. This, as we discussed in Chapter 8, is dangerous for children too. Children need these toys and equipment, but often there are more lying around than the children are using at any one time. Keeping floor areas clear reduces hazards. Children's independence and self-help skills are also encouraged when they are involved in tidying up.

Areas which are used as thoroughfares must always be kept clear, with no pushers, prams or bags lying round. Not only does this prevent staff, parents and children tripping over, a necessary exit is clear in the case of fire and emergency evacuation.

Child care also means spills. There are spills from the drinks at snack and meal times, there are spills in the painting area, in the home corner where cups of tea are being made. Spills should be wiped up immediately and it helps to use a floor cover which can be easily washed and dried.

Staff can also help reduce falls, trips and slips by wearing appropriate clothing and footwear. Non-slip, flat-heeled, covered shoes are comfortable and safe. Comfortable clothes such as jeans and t-shirts allow for movement with no trailing sleeves or skirts to get caught on equipment or to cause tripping.

Lifting and manual handling

Lifting is part of child care but hazards can be minimised by examining alternatives to lifting.

- A toddler can walk to a change table rather than being carried. Steps can be made so that the child can climb onto the change table with assistance.
- Staff can kneel on the floor to comfort a distressed child rather than pick the child up.
- Use of linen carriers and other carrying equipment on wheels avoids having to lift.

Where lifting is unavoidable, then the correct techniques must be used. It is part of an employer's responsibility to ensure that all staff (including relief staff) know how to lift with a straight body and back, and bent knees.

Employers can also help prevent lifting injuries by providing equipment that is easy to use. A change table should be high enough to allow a baby to be changed without the staff member having to stoop down. Storage shelves should be easily reached without stretching or bending.

There should also be rules about lifting equipment and the number of people needed for safe lifting practice.

Staff equipment

Equipment such as tables and chairs used by staff should be well designed and sturdy. When possible, staff should sit in an adult-sized chair. Some children's services have 'teachers' chairs' which are larger than a child's chair but still allow an adult to be at the physical level of the children.

Chemicals

Frequently used chemicals in child care are chlorine-based and these are very dangerous if inhaled. Bleach is used for cleaning and needs to be diluted. Gloves should be worn at all times when handling bleach.

Chlorine will be used if there is a wading or swimming pool in the service. The fumes from powdered chlorine are extremely dangerous. It is best however to use liquid chlorine and this will prevent burns from undissolved powder. Only small amounts will be needed to chlorinate a wading pool but extreme care must be taken. Gloves must be worn and any spills onto skin immediately washed off with plenty of cold water.

Some wooden equipment, especially outdoor equipment, is treated with chemicals so that it withstands the weather. The chemicals used should be checked for safety before purchase.

A Material Safety Data Sheet should be supplied by manufacturers for ALL chemical substances. This includes information about what chemicals make up the substance, how to handle, how to store as well as vital first aid information.

Electricity

Electricity, which is used in all aspects of our work and home lives, is fatal if handled wrongly. All electrical equipment should be maintained in excellent order. Where possible, all power points should be of the type that automatically switch off if anything but a proper plug is inserted. Some older buildings do not have these plugs, and power point protectors should be used.

Emergency situations

Fire

Legislation requires that all efforts are made to prevent fire. Fire protection equipment such as alarms, fire extinguishers, fire mats/blankets (near stoves), smoke alarms must be in place at all times and tested on a regular basis. Most equipment is checked to see it is in working order every 12 months.

Fire drills should be carried out at least every four months. This includes practising evacuation procedures.

Bomb scare

This is another situation where all staff and children might need to be evacuated from the centre.

Where possible, in the case of a bomb scare, attempts should be made to keep the caller on the phone. Another staff member should immediately call the police on another phone (mobiles are useful here) and raise the alarm in the centre. The staff person taking the call should note as much about the caller as possible such as gender, accent, type of voice, background noises. This may help the police identify a suspect or a place from where the call was made.

Emergency evacuation

The ease of evacuation depends on routine ongoing safety measures.

- All exits should be kept free of equipment and furniture at all times.
- Keys to any locked doors must be carried by staff members at all times.
- Loose flammable rubbish should not be left lying around. The storage rooms in children's services often contain 'junk' material being kept for collage and other art activities.
- All staff should be trained in the use of all fire-fighting equipment.
- Attendance sheets should be easily accessible

Evacuation procedures

The service should have nominated at least two safe assembly areas away from the centre which are large enough to accommodate all children and staff. Previous planning should ensure that individual staff members are allocated tasks to:

- Raise alarm within the service.
- Report the emergency, note and carry out advice from emergency personnel.

- Collect roll/attendance sheet and first aid kit.
- Assist with evacuation of mobile children.
- Assist with the evacuation of immobile children—eg. babies and those children with special needs. This procedure ought to be planned well beforehand and practised during fire drill. Several babies can be evacuated in one cot but staff must check beforehand that the cot fits easily through all doors.
- Check areas such as storerooms and toilets.
- Using the attendance sheet, check that all children and staff are at the assembly area.
- Immediately give names of those not there to emergency workers.
- Calm and reassure children.
- Follow the orders of the emergency workers.

It is important that each children's service have a list of emergency procedures highlighted in appropriate places. This includes emergency phone numbers for fire, police and ambulance.

Working together to provide health and safety in the workplace

Occupational health and safety can be best achieved by all persons and organisations working together. This includes government organisations, trade unions and professional organisations, management, workers and parents.

Co-operation is needed at the official level of legislation and it is important in the workplace. Identifying work-based problems and finding positive solutions needs much effort and good will from all persons in the workplace.

Learning activities

1. Find out about the occupational health and safety legislation in your State or Territory. Who administers Workers' Compensation?
2. Check the immunisation requirements and recommendations for staff in your State or Territory. Are you up to date with your own immunisation?
3. In the scenario about Kay, identify the stresses that she has experienced in the first two hours of work this Monday morning.
4. How does Kay reduce the stress caused by her job? What are some of your activities which help to reduce stress?

Reference

Mathews J. (1985). *Health and safety at work*. Sydney, Pluto Press.

Further reading

Many States and Territories have Occupational Health and Safety publications relating especially to children's services.

An example is:

WorkCover Authority. (1994). *WorkCover child care information, New South Wales.*

CHAPTER 12

Community health resources for child care

WE HAVE EMPHASISED throughout this book how child care is part of community health services. Child-care professionals are an integral part of the health team responsible for the wellbeing of children. Child care often provides the link between children, families and other health professionals. Children's services are also a health resource for parents who feel comfortable voicing concerns in a familiar environment with familiar staff who know and understand their child.

This responsibility means that caregivers need to have an understanding of the health services available to children and parents. There are many services available which are provided by a combination of Commonwealth, State or Territory, and Local governments. Non-government organisations also play a role, giving support to families with specific needs, for instance, Asthma Australia. See Tables 12.1, 12.2, 12.3 and 12.4.

Commonwealth Government

Funds for health care in Australia come from the Commonwealth Government through the Department of Health and Aged Care. The Commonwealth Department of Family and Community Services promotes programs which support families. States and Territories allocate their own funds, as well as Commonwealth funds from these departments to run their health and family services programs.

The Commonwealth Government directly funds immunisation programs throughout Australia. State and Territory governments are responsible for organising immunisation sessions and for allocating funds to other health services.

Other agencies that are funded through the Commonwealth Government include:

- The National Health and Medical Research Council
- The Australian Institute of Health and Welfare.
  (see Appendix 2)

The Department of Family and Community Services is responsible for Children's Services which includes accreditation procedures through the Quality Improvement and Accreditation System. The Child Care Benefit scheme is administered through this department.

Table 12.1. Commonweath Government services

Commonwealth Department	Contact web address
Department of Health and Aged Care	*www.health.gov.au* htttp://pilot.healthinsite.gov.au This second website is part of the Department of Health and Aged Care. It contains a wide range of relevant health information including child health.
Department of Family and Community Services	*www.facs.gov.au* Within this site, there is a Childcare Program section with valuable up-to-date information on current issues in children's services.

State and Territory governments

These governments are responsible for the management and delivery of many health services. In some areas the Local Government Councils may be involved in community health.

Family and child health services

These services are offered in each State and Territory. They may be part of a Community Health Centre or be a separate service. They may be named Maternal and Child Health Centres, though they would generally include care for all the family.

Family and child health services play an important role in preventing health problems and maintaining health. Infants and young children are weighed, measured and checked for developmental milestones. Immunisation is given and general health assessed.

Health screening at pre-school or school entry level is also carried out by this service (see Surveillance and Screening in Chapter 4). Parental concerns are noted and discussed. Referrals to other services and allied health professionals are arranged if there is concern for the health of a child.

Table 12.2. State and Territory services

State Department	Contact web address
New South Wales Department of Health	*www.health.nsw.gov.au*
Queensland Department of Health	*www.health.qld.gov.au*
South Australian Department of Human Services Community, family, health and housing	*www.health.sa.gov.au*
Department of Health and Human Service Tasmania	*www.dchs.tas.gov.au*
Department of Human Services A Victorian State Government Department	*www.dhs.vic.gov.au*
Health Department of Western Australia	*www.health.wa.gov.au*
Health ACT (Australian Capital Territory)	*www.health.act.gov.au*
Territory Health Services (Northern Territory)	*www.nt.gov.au/nths*

Non-government organisations

Many of these groups started as support groups for parents and have developed into organisations which provide health education and promote research. These organisations generally do not receive government funding though they may be awarded research grants. Administrative staff are usually employed, with volunteers doing other work including fund raising. An example of how this works is Red Nose Day, which raises funds for SIDSaustralia.

The following table gives an example of the many non-government organisations linked to child health. The contact details of the State and Territory branches can be obtained from the national website.

Table 12.3. Non-government support organisations

Organisation name	Aims of organisation	Contacts
National Asthma Campaign	To: • Improve the quality of life and health outcomes of people with asthma and their carers • Reduce the social and economic impact of asthma on the community • Reduce the prevalence	National Asthma Campaign (Aus) 1 Palmerston Crescent South Melbourne Vic 3205 Phone 03 9214 1476 Fax 03 9214 1400 *nac@nationalasthma.org.au* *www.NationalAsthma.org.au*
Asthma Australia	To eliminate asthma as a major cause of ill health and disruption in the community. Asthma Associations and Foundations in each State and Territory offer educational services to child care staff and families.	Addresses for all State and Territory Asthma Foundations can be obtained from: Phone 1800 645 130 and *www.asthmaaustralia.org.au*
Diabetes Australia	Is a federation of 12 major diabetes organisations. Major aims are: • To promote and fund research into all aspects of diabetes • To improve the quality of life and assistance provided to those affected by diabetes • To increasse the public awareness of the disease.	National office: 218 Northbourne Ave Braddon ACT Phone 02 6230 1155 Fax 02 6230 1535 *www.diabetesaustralia.com.au* Divisions in all States and Territories

Continued

Table 12.3. (*Continued*)

Organisation name	**Aims of organisation**	**Contacts**
National Association for the Prevention of Child Abuse and Neglect (NAPCAN)	Aims to work for the prevention of all forms of child abuse—child abuse being defined as: anything which individuals, institutions or processes do, or fail to do, which directly or indirectly harms children or damages their prospects of a safe and healthy development into adulthood.	NAPCAN Australia Office: Suite 3 8-24 Kippax Street Surrey Hills NSW 2010 Phone 02 9211 0224 Fax 02 9211 5676 *napcanaus@aol.com* *www.napcan.org.au*
Nursing Mothers' Association of Australia	To provide factual information for all women to make informed choices about feeding their babies and their parenting styles. To be active participants in government enquiries and committees concerning breastfeeding. To give women confidence in themselves as women and mothers. To create an awareness in the community of the importance of human milk, breastfeeding and nurturing. To work with health professionals and others in the community to provide an optimum environment for women to establish and continue breastfeeding.	National headquarters: 18118-1822 Malvern Rd Malvern, Victoria PO Box 4000 Glen Iris Vic 3146 Ph 03 9885 0855 Fax 03 9885 0866 *nursingm@nmaa.asn.au* *http://avoca.vicnet.net.au/~nmaa/nmaa/index.html* There are Helplines in all States and Territories which can be contacted via the main site.

SIDSaustralia	Provides a wide range of family programs including grief and bereavement counselling, health promotion and education assisting the families of children aged six years and under who die suddenly and unexpectedly regardless of cause. Promotes research into SIDS.	National Office: National SIDS Council of Australia Level 1 891 Burke Road Camberwell Victoria 3124 Phone 03 9813 3200 Fax 03 9813 3099 *national@sidsaustralia.org.au* *http//:www.sidsaustralia.org.au*
Kidsafe Australia (Child Accident Prevention Foundation of Australia)	Is an independent non-profit organisation dedicated to preventing accidental death and injury in children. Works at a national, state and local level and in cooperation with government, industry, schools, hospitals, the media, community groups, voluntary organisations and individuals. Conducts public education campaigns, provides information, develops resources and initiates special projects to lift awareness of child safety issues and injury prevention.	National Office: Level 1 224 Church Street Richmond Victoria Phone 03 9427 1008 Fax 03 9421 3831 *Kidsafe@greenweb.com.au* *http://www.greenweb.com.au.kidsafe* There are Divisions of Kidsafe in each State and Territory. Some States have Safe Homes which display safe equipment and furniture.

Table 12.3. (*Continued*)

Organisation name	**Aims of organisation**	**Contacts**
Association for the Welfare of Children in Hospital (AWCH)	AWCH is a national not-for-profit community organisation of concerned parents, health professionals, and community members, who work together to ensure the emotional and social needs of children and adolescents are recognised and met within hospitals and health care systems in Australia.	National Office: PO Box 113 Westmead NSW 2145 Phone 02 9633 1988 Fax 02 9633 1180 *awch@enternet.com.au*

Table 12.4. Research organisations
There are many research groups working to improve the health and welfare of children and their families. Many of these groups are attached to universities; others are established as research institutes.

Name	Role	Contact
Australian Institute of Family Studies	Is an independent statutory authority which was established in 1980 to promote the identification and understanding of factors affecting marital and family stability in Australia. The Institute is linked through the Commonwealth Government to the Department of Family and Community Services.	300 Queen Street Melbourne Victoria 3000 Phone 03 9214 7888 Fax 03 9214 7839 *http://www.aifs.org.au* *webmaster@aifs.org.au*
National Child Protection Clearing House	Is located at the Institute of Family Studies. Is funded by the Department of Family and Community Services under the auspices of the National Child Protection Council as part of the national strategy for the prevention of child abuse and neglect. Research papers and reports can be obtained from the Clearing House.	Is found on the main Institute for Family Studies website.
TVW Telethon Institute for Child Health Research	Is committed to investigating the causes of childhood diseases, particularly those which cause the most anguish and cost to families and the community. Major research programs are: • Asthma • Maternal and child health • Childhood leukaemia and cancer research • Psychosocial research.	TVW Telethon Institute for Child Health Research PO Box 855 West Perth Western Australia 6872 Phone 08 9489 777 Fax 08 9489 7700 *http://www.ichr.uwa.edu.au* *enquire@ichr.uwa.edu.au*

General practitioners

General practitioners are usually the first medical service a family attends when seeking health advice. Traditionally known as the family doctor, the general practitioner of old often cared for the health of a person from birth to death. While families (and doctors) move more these days, the contemporary family doctor cares for the whole person and their family. General practitioners offer immunisation services and also emphasise the prevention of disease as well as the treatment of illness.

Many general practitioners continue training after finishing medical school and are admitted to the Royal Australasian College of General Practitioners. The College offers ongoing education so doctors can keep up to date with advances in preventive medicine and treatments.

The health care system in Australia is mainly government funded, with payment to general practitioners for patient services being controlled by the Commonwealth Government through Medicare. Individual general practitioners and group practices may bulk bill the government for all services so patients do not pay for visits to the doctor. Most general practitioners, however, charge more than the scheduled Medicare fee and patients need to pay the gap amount personally. There is an agreement that those persons who are economically disadvantaged and hold a health care card will not have to pay more than the Medicare fee.

Each geographical area in Australia has a Division of General Practice whose role is to encourage interaction between general practitioners, government, health authorities, other health professionals and the community.

Paediatricians

The word 'paedi' is derived from the Greek work for a child. Paediatricians are child health specialists who have taken special intensive training over several years and passed examinations which admit them to the Royal Australasian College of Physicians.

Children with special health needs will be referred to a paediatrician by a general practitioner. Paediatricians work from private specialist rooms or may be seen in an out-patients clinic at a hospital.

Children's hospitals

Most States have specialist children's hospitals which are sometimes administered in combination with a women's hospital. The large children's hospitals are centres of excellence not only for the specialised treatment of children, but also for parent support and education, and research into child health. These hospitals, which are usually associated with a university medical school, are also responsible for the education of undergraduate medical students, trainee paediatricians, nurses and allied health professionals. These are known as teaching hospitals (see Table 12.5). Parent information and education is part of the role of these hospitals and many have health education material on their websites.

In places where there is not a children's hospital, there are specialist paediatric wards within public hospitals. Large private hospitals also have specialist paediatric wards. Many of the teaching hospitals are members of the Australian Association of Paediatric Teaching Centres.

Table 12.5. Australian paediatric teaching hospitals

State/Territory	**Hospital**	**Contact** Some hospitals are accessed through the State/Territory Health Department
Australian Capital Territory	The Canberra Hospital	*www.canberrahospital.act.gov.au*
New South Wales	The New Children's Hospital, Sydney Sydney Children's Hospital John Hunter Children's Hospital, Newcastle	*www.nch.edu.au* *www.sch.edu.au* *www.hunter.health.nsw.gov.au*
Northern Territory	Royal Darwin Hospital	*www.nt.gov.au/nths/royal darwinhospital*
Queensland	Mater Misericordiae Children's Hospital, Brisbane Royal Children's Hospital, Brisbane	*www.mater.org.au* *www.health.qld.gov.au*
South Australia	Flinders Medical Centre, Adelaide Women's and Children's Hospital, Adelaide	*www.flinders.sa.gov.au* *www.wch.sa.gov.au*
Tasmania	Royal Hobart Hospital	*www.dchs.tas.gov.au*
Victoria Victoria	Monash Medical Centre, Melbourne Royal Children's Hospital, Melbourne	*www.med.monash.edu.au* *www.rch.unimelb.edu.au*
Western Australia	Princess Margaret Hospital for Children, Perth	*www.pmh.wa.gov.au*

Allied health and other professionals

There are many other groups of workers whose role is crucial to child health. Allied health professionals are involved in many aspects of child care and development including early intervention and special needs programs. The input of an allied health professional is often needed for the successful integration of children with special needs into mainstream children's services.

Dietitians

The family of a child who has a condition where a special diet is needed (eg. diabetes, phenylketonuria) will have the support of a community dietitian. The dietician will discuss the family and cultural food preferences and develop lists of foods the child is able to eat. Explanations and information about the reasons for the special diet are also given. There may also be help with menu planning.

Community dietitians are used by many child-care centres when planning general menus as well as special diets (see Chapter 7).

Occupational therapists

The occupational therapist is concerned with the creative adaptation of equipment and toys so that a disabled or injured child can have the same learning experiences as other children. The occupational therapist also plans activities which increase a child's skills and helps an injured child to recover fullest possible capacity.

There are many situations where occupational therapists work with children. A child who has special physical needs may need feeding equipment to be adapted so that he is able to feed himself and thus have independence.

Physiotherapists

This group of allied health professionals are concerned with muscle function and movement. A physiotherapist may devise some developmentally appropriate exercises and games to assist a disabled or injured child to walk or improve mobility and limb movement. Child-care staff and parents will learn how to carry out these exercises and games. Physiotherapists and occupational therapists often work closely together in early intervention programs as well as in the care of the child with a temporary injury or long-term special needs.

Speech pathologists

Some children have difficulty in speaking due to the physical structure of their mouth as when the mouth is not fully formed. Other children, such as those with cerebral palsy, have muscle movement problems and find it difficult to form sounds. A speech therapist would work intensely with these children. Children who are hearing-impaired will also have speech problems and would be referred to a speech pathologist.

Audiologists

Children who are suspected of having a degree of hearing impairment would have their hearing assessed by an audiologist. There are many highly technical ways of measuring the type and amount of hearing loss and of trying to minimise the loss through the wearing of hearing aids. Audiologists and speech pathologists work very closely together.

Psychologists

Psychologists are non-medical people who are trained in behavioural science. This is distinct from psychiatrists who are medically trained in mental health and illness. The two professions often work together.

Psychologists will work with children who have behavioural problems. Working with the whole family is usually important too. Some psychologists work as counsellors and give family (and staff) support in times of crisis as well as being available for ongoing support.

Social workers

Social workers have particular skills in counselling. They are trained to care for the social needs of families and others within our community. Social needs are frequently linked to economic needs and social workers often help arrange for financial support from government and other agencies.

Dental therapists

One of the roles of the dental therapist is that of early childhood dental education. This dental education might be done with an individual child in a dentist's surgery or with groups of children in child care and preschool. The habits of lifelong dental hygiene are set when young so this is an important part of preventive health.

Community pharmacists

Pharmacists dispense medicines that have been prescribed by a medical practitioner (see Chapter 10). It is the pharmacist who ensures that families understand how and when to give the medicine, so they have an important educative role. Pharmacies also sell many patent medicines and can give advice regarding the use of such products as teething gel, infant pain relievers and vitamins. Health education material is found in pharmacies and is therefore very accessible to families.

Other allied health professions

- Orthoptics: the development of eye muscle exercises for conditions such as squint so that straight vision is achieved.
- Orthotics: the use of braces and other splints to achieve a straight body.
- Podiatry: the diagnosing and treating of disorders of the feet.
- Prosthetics: the making and fitting of artificial parts of the body such as limbs and eyes.

Putting it all together

The complex array of health services can be quite daunting. Even health professionals get confused at times, especially when the names and types of services change. This chapter has tried to give an overview of health resources and services within the Australian system in order to help you understand what is available and how it all fits together.

APPENDIX 1

Links between chapter contents and the National Child Care Competency Standards

Chapters	National competency standards
Chapter 1: Introduction to health	CHCCD3A Meet information needs of the community CHCORG3A Participate in the work environment CHCRF1A Communicate with family members about their child CHCCN20A Advocate for the rights and needs of children
Chapter 2: Choosing to have children	CHCCD3A Meet information needs of the community CHCCD7A Support community resources
Chapter 3: Having children	CHCCNAA Support babies' needs CHCCN5A Support the emotional wellbeing of babies/infants
Chapter 4: The growing and developing child	CHCCN2A Provide physical care CHCICAA Communicate with children CHCFC1A Support the development of children in the service CC1C1A Interact positively with children CHCICAA Communicate with children CHCFC2A Foster the physical development of children CHCFC3A Foster the social development of children

Chapters	National competency standards
	CHCFC4A Foster the emotional and psychological development of children CHCFC5A Foster children's cognitive development CHCRF1A Communicate with family members about their child CHCCNAA Support babies' needs
Chapter 5: Infectious diseases	CHCCHILD1A Work within legislative requirements CHCCOM1A Communicate with people accessing the services of the organisation
Chapter 6: Hygiene practices and health routines	CHCCN1A Maintain a healthy and safe environment CHCCN7A Foster children's self-help skills CHCPR2A Organise experiences for children CHCCN8A Plan care routines CHCFC6A Foster children's language development CHCCN2A Provide physical care CHCCN10A Support the emotional needs of children CHCIC1A Interact positively with children CHCIC4A Work collaboratively with children
Chapter 7: Nutrition	CHCCN3A Prepare food CHCFC1A Support the development of children in the service CHCFC6A Foster children's language development
Chapter 8: Child safety	CHCCN4A Respond to illness, accidents and emergencies CHCCN6A Travel with children safely CHCCN11A Guide the establishment and maintenance of a safe environment

Chapters	National competency standards
Chapter 9: Child protection	CHCCHILD2A Support the rights and safety of children within duty-of-care requirements CHCCILC1A Work within legislative and ethical requirements CHCCN11A Guide the establishment and maintenance of a safe environment CHCPR9A Use observations and records
Chapter 10: Illness in child care	CHCCN4A Respond to illness, accidents and emergencies CHCRF1A Communicate with family members about their children CHCPR9A Use observations and records CHCF11A Work in partnership with families to care for the child
Chapter 11: Occupational health and safety	CHCORG4A Follow the organisation's occupational health and safety policies
Chapter 12: Community health resources for child care	CHCC3DA Meet information needs of the community

APPENDIX 2

Organisations and agencies

Australian Early Childhood Association (AECA) is a non-profit organisation that acts in the interests of children from birth to eight years of age and for older children in care outside of schools hours. It actively promotes the provision of high-quality services for all young children and their families. AECA publishes specialist literature on early childhood in the form of the *Every Child* magazine, booklets in the *Research in Practice* series and the *Australian Journal of Early Childhood.*

Australian Health Ministers' Advisory Council (AHMAC) advises Commonwealth, State and Territory Government Ministers of Health. This group decides on policy matters that affect the health of all Australians. For example, in 1995 AHMAC published a national health policy for children and young people: *The Health of Young Australians.*

Australian Institute of Health and Welfare is Australia's national health and welfare statistics and information agency and is part of the Commonwealth Government's Health and Aged Care portfolio. The Institute's mission is to improve the health and well-being of Australians by informing community discussion and decision-making through national leadership in developing and providing health and welfare statistics and information. Institute publications include *Australia's Health 2000* and *Australia's Children 1998: Their health and wellbeing.*

The National Gowrie/RAP (Resource and Advisory Program) Consortium promotes better practice in children's services through professional advice, support and training. There is a Lady Gowrie Child Care Centre in each State capital city. The Centres provide a range of programs to support professionals working in children's services, such as training and access to resource centres.

National Health and Medical Research Council (NHMRC) is a Commonwealth Government agency that is committed to raising the standard of individual and public health in Australia. NHMRC sponsors many health publications, eg. *Staying Healthy in Child Care*. It develops many policies on health and publishes guidelines such as *Dietary guidelines for children and adolescents* and the recommended immunisation schedule. NHMRC is the major source of medical research funding within Australia.

Quality Improvement and Accreditation System (QIAS) was set up to ensure that children in long-day care centres have stimulating, positive experiences and interactions which will foster all aspects of their development. QIAS oversees the accreditation of long-day care centres throughout Australia. To become accredited, a centre must meet the standards laid down in the Principles of the National Childcare Accreditation Council. This council also administers the scheme through the Commonwealth Government. The accreditation status of a child-care centre is evidence of the standard of care offered to families.

World Health Organization (WHO), an agency of the United Nations, works in an advisory, educative and technical role with governments and health agencies all around the world. Its main objective is to assist all peoples in the world to attain the highest possible level of health.

GLOSSARY OF TERMS

Active immunity occurs when the body makes its own antibodies against the antigens of a disease. This happens when the a baby (or older person) is immunised against the disease or when an unimmunised person gets the disease.

Antibodies are substances which are made by the body to fight the antigens from germs. Specific antibodies are made against specific antigens.

Antigens are the substances made by specific germs or micro-organisms. Each germ can make a number of different antigens which can contribute to the child getting sick. Some antigens, such as whooping cough toxin, are harmful to the body and make the illness worse.

Areas of development (sometimes referred to as domains of development)
Physical development includes growth and movement (motor).

- gross motor refers to the large movements such as sitting up, rolling, crawling, walking, climbing.
- fine motor refers to small movements such as moving the eyes, smiling, picking up small objects with the fingers, drawing and writing.

Intellectual development includes:

- gaining language—the babbling and gooing noises made by young babies are part of language development in the pre-verbal stage.
- cognitive skills, which are those of thinking, remembering, reasoning and solving problems.

Emotional (psychological) development is the way the child makes close bonds with people who are important to the child.

Social development is the way the child learns to get on with other children and adults.

Blended families is a term applied to families which are made up of children, step-children and half-siblings. A common blended family of today is where each parent has previously had children with another partner and also with each other.

- Sibling is a brother or sister with the same two parents.
- Half-sibling is a brother or sister of one parent only.
- Step-sibling is a child of a new partner of the mother or father.

Body defences are the built-in ways the body fights the germs that can invade the body and cause disease.

Chromosomes are the structures which carry all the genes. There are 23 pairs of chromosomes in the nucleus of each cell in the human body.

Cross-infection is the transmission of infection from one person to another. This can happen in many ways, which are described in Chapter 5.

Developmental assessment looks to see whether a child's developmental progress is within the normal range. Any concerns can be noted and referred to a specialist in that area of development to seek advice about the need for early intervention programs.

Developmental delay is the term used when a child is not reaching the normal developmental milestones in an area (or areas) of development. The child would have been formally assessed for this situation to be recognised (see Early intervention).

Developmental regression is when a child has reached a certain stage of development (see Milestones) and then goes back to an earlier stage. This can happen for no obvious reason but often occurs with 2 to 3 year olds after the birth of a brother or sister, or some other event which is upsetting for the child. A child who was dry during the day may start to need to wear nappies again or may want to return to a bottle for drinking. (see Sibling adjustment in Chapter 3).

Diet is the food we habitually eat. Some people may be on a special diet for weight loss or to control a disease such as diabetes. Most children and adults do not require a special diet but one which contains all the necessary nutrients for that person's stage of life and level of activity.

Disinfectants are substances which kill or inactivate large numbers of germs. Disinfectants will not eliminate all germs but, used properly on surfaces that have already been cleaned, they should bring the number of germs down to an acceptable level.

The two main disinfectants used in child care are:

- Quaternary compounds (quats) which are common household disinfectants. Quats kill some bacteria but not viruses.
- Bleach, which is capable of killing most germs. It is relatively inexpensive but needs to be handled carefully and diluted according to instructions, for use. Bleach is corrosive to metal objects and fades colours from clothes.

Early intervention is the term applied to any special treatment or programs which aim to overcome any type of developmental delay in young children. These programs may also need to find ways that will help the child to make up or compensate for the delay.

Embryo is the term by which the fertilised human egg (ovum) is known until it is 8 weeks old.

Endemic describes a particular disease when it is present in a community all the time.

Epidemic describes the situation when there are several cases of a particular infectious disease in a community at a particular time, but not at other times.

Exclusion period is the time that a person with a particular disease is likely to infect others and therefore must stay away from child care, school, work or other public places.

Fetus is the term used for a prenatal baby from 8 weeks after fertilisation until birth.

Heterozygous is where the two genes (one from the mother and one from the father) for a given characteristic, such as blood group, are different. One gene may be dominant and the other hidden or recessive.

Homozygous is where the two genes (one from each parent) for a given characteristic, such as blood group, are the same (Chapter 3).

Immunisation (vaccination) is when a small controlled amount of a substance containing antigens (with any toxins neutralised) from a specific germ is put into the body. This prompts the body to make antibodies without getting sick from the disease. These antibodies will then help to protect the person from ever getting the disease.

Incubation period is the time between when a germ first enters the body and the first signs or symptom occurring. Incubation periods can vary from a few days (eg. common cold) to many years (eg. AIDS).

***In vitro* fertilisation** means the fertilisation of a female ovum by a male sperm outside of the body. Female eggs and male sperm are collected and brought together in a dish, where fertilisation takes place. The fertilised egg is then placed into the female uterus. (*In vitro* means 'in glass' but today most laboratory workers actually use plastic dishes.)

Infectious (communicable) diseases are diseases caused by micro-organisms (germs) that can be transmitted from one person to another. This transmission can happen in many ways, as described in Chapter 5.

Kilojoules (calories) are the measure of how much energy is in particular food. A very small amount of food high in fat, such as chocolate, has the same amount of energy (number of kilojoules) as larger amounts of fruit and vegetables.

Mandatory reporting in a child-care context is a legal requirement that all suspected instances of child abuse shall be reported to the appropriate authorities.

Micro-organisms are too small to be seen with the naked eye. Some micro-organisms cause disease and are commonly called germs.

Milestones are developmental changes that are noted as a sign of the developmental changes in the child. Some milestones in the first two years include smiling, rolling over, sitting up unaided, crawling, first words, walking.

Non-prescribed medication can be purchased without a prescription from a chemist, health food store or supermarket. Mild analgesics such as paracetomol as well as vitamins and herbal medicine come into this category.

Nutrients are protein, fat, carbohydrates, minerals and vitamins found in food. The body needs particular nutrients for growth and the healthy functioning of all tissues and body systems. Too much or too little of a particular nutrient can cause harm to the body and health of a person.

Passive immunity is when a person has received antibodies against a specific disease (or diseases). Babies may receive maternal antibodies from their mother *in utero* and also through breast milk. This passive immunity helps to protect the baby from infections for the first few months of life.

Peers are people or groups of people with similar interests or skills or stages of development. A child caregiver's peer group could be her colleagues, a child's peers could be the other children in his group or children the same age.

Percentile growth charts are used to assess the growth of an individual child and compare it with that of all Australian children of the same age and gender. Percentile charts are available for traits such as height, weight and head circumference.

Prescribed medication is that which is prescribed by a registered medical practitioner and dispensed by a registered pharmacist. A prescription is needed for this medication to be dispensed. The medication will be clearly marked with the name of the drug and the strength of the drug as well as the patient's name, the amount to be taken and how often it is to be taken.

Psittacosis is a respiratory disease that can be transmitted from birds to humans.

Psychosocial skills refers to a person's ability to have close emotional relationships with those who are important in their lives and also to be able to have positive relationships with the many others with whom the person comes into contact.

Setting limits provides guidance for children regarding safe and acceptable behaviour. The way limits are set depends on the stage of development of the child. Toddlers need an environment where there is adequate space, equipment and attention from caring adults. Older children still need attention but are able to understand rules and directions as to what is acceptable behaviour.

Structure and function of body systems may also be described as anatomy and physiology of the human body. Structure or anatomy gives information about what organs, tissues and cells make up the body system. Function or physiology describes what the structures do, or how they work together to form a body system.

Theories on child development are explanations of how and why changes in growth, movement, language, thinking and relationships occur in children as they move from infancy to toddlerhood through preschool and middle childhood to adolescence. These theories are mainly formed by psychologists who have studied certain aspects of child development, often over several years. New theories are suggested as new information about children is discovered. Some early theorists were Freud, Piaget, Gesell. Some more recent theorists are Vygotsky, Brofenbrenner, Belsky.

Toxoplasmosis is a disease which can be spread by germs in animal faeces. It is particularly dangerous in pregnant women as it can cause intellectual and physical disability in the unborn child.

Ultrasound is a test which uses high pitched sound waves to find out the size and shape of any structure within the body. It is used in pregnancy to see how big the fetus is and if there are any concerns about fetal development. Ultrasound was done only if there were concerns about the fetus, but it has now become a routine test. However, the test may be done in future only when there are specific concerns about size and development.

INDEX